W9-CFS-159

Recent Advances in
PSORIASIS
The Role of the Immune System

Barbara S Baker

Imperial College School of Medicine at St Mary's, London

Recent Advances in
PSORIASIS
The Role of the
Immune System

Imperial College Press

Published by

Imperial College Press
57 Shelton Street
Covent Garden
London WC2H 9HE

Distributed by

World Scientific Publishing Co. Pte. Ltd.
P O Box 128, Farrer Road, Singapore 912805
USA office: Suite 1B, 1060 Main Street, River Edge, NJ 07661
UK office: 57 Shelton Street, Covent Garden, London WC2H 9HE

British Library Cataloguing-in-Publication Data
A catalogue record for this book is available from the British Library.

RECENT ADVANCES IN PSORIASIS: THE ROLE OF THE IMMUNE SYSTEM

ISBN   1-86094-120-6

This book is printed on acid and chlorine free paper.

Printed in Singapore by FuIsland Offset Printing

Preface

Psoriasis is considered as a disease of epidermal hyperproliferation induced by T lymphocytes. The purpose of this book is to bring together the various pieces of evidence that have contributed to our current understanding of the role of the immune system in psoriasis. The latest approaches to investigating the immunopathogenesis of this disease, and a review of previous findings, are presented to give an overall picture of the current knowledge in this field. Novel therapies to treat this disease are described, some of which are already being tested on patients. Unlike current treatments, these new approaches have the potential to switch off the disease process on a long-term basis. In addition, a model is proposed for the immunopathogenesis of psoriasis which hopefully will serve as a basis for further research.

The findings presented here illustrate the considerable progress that has been been achieved in recent years in our understanding of the immunopathogenic mechanisms involved in this common skin disease.

I would like to thank Professor Lionel Fry with whom I have collaborated on this work over a period of almost 20 years, and who continues to give me support and encouragement.

Barbara S. Baker
Imperial College School of
Medicine at St. Mary's
London

Contents

CHAPTER 1

Aetiology, Clinical and Histological Features of Psoriasis

1.1 Clinical Features

Psoriasis is a chronic, inflammatory skin disease affecting approximately 2% of Caucasians. A seronegative arthropathy is present in 6–30%[1,2] of patients, and both Crohn's disease and ulcerative colitis show a positive association.[3] The onset of the disease can occur at any age but is more frequent around puberty. Two further peaks of increased frequency have also been observed at about 30 and 50 years of age, but there is a considerable overlap between the three groups.[4]

The typical psoriatic lesion is a raised red scaly patch with a sharply demarcated edge. In chronic plaque (CP) psoriasis, the commonest form of the disease, the plaques characteristically occur on the the extensor surfaces of the knees and elbows, scalp and sacral region (Fig. 1.1). In contrast, the lesions of guttate psoriasis are smaller and occur over the upper trunk. The limbs, face and scalp may also be affected (Fig. 1.2). Guttate psoriasis typically appears 1–2 weeks after a streptococcal upper respiratory tract infection in children and young adults and, unlike CP psoriasis, often spontaneously resolves after 8–12 weeks. Around 60–70% of patients with guttate psoriasis develop the chronic form of the disease at a later date[5] suggesting that the two clinical types are linked by common factors. Other less frequently observed forms of psoriasis include erythrodermic (100% involvement

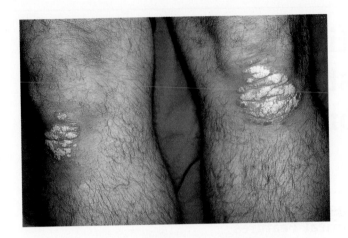

Fig. 1.1. Chronic plaque psoriasis.

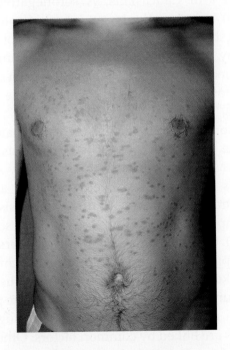

Fig. 1.2. Guttate psoriasis.

of skin) and pustular psoriasis whose pathogenesis has not been widely studied and therefore will not be discussed here.

1.2 Genetics

1.2.1 *Epidemiology*

Strong evidence for a genetic basis for psoriasis was first provided by two large-scale epidemiological studies in the Faroe Islands[6] and Sweden[7] which revealed significantly higher incidences of psoriasis in relatives compared to the general population, or to matched controls. Thus, the risk to first degree relatives was estimated to be 8–23% and the prevalence of psoriasis 2–2.8% in the study populations as a whole.[6,7] Re-examination of the data from these two studies by Elder *et al.*[8] demonstrated that the data was consistent with a multilocus model of inheritance.

Further evidence for the involvement of genetic factors in psoriasis was suggested by twin studies which showed that the concordance in monozygotic twins was 63–70%[9,10] compared to 23% in dizygotic twins.[10] In both studies, the age of onset of the disease and its manifestations were very similar in the concordant monozygotic twins.[9,10] Since the concordance rates are not 100%, environmental factors are implicated in the triggering of the disease (Sec. 1.3).

1.2.2 *Mode of Inheritance*

The mode of inheritance in psoriasis remains unclear with reports of both autosomal dominant[11] and recessive[12] patterns of inheritance in families. However, much of the available data concerning the frequency of psoriasis in siblings with neither, one or both parents affected with the disease do not appear to fit either model even after taking into account age-dependent penetrance.[13]

The consensus appears to be that the data is most consistent with a polygenic or multifactorial pattern of inheritance, the latter including the involvement of environmental factors.

1.2.3 *Genomic Imprinting*

The term "genomic imprinting" refers to a differential expression/ activity of a gene depending on whether it has been inherited from the mother or father. Genomic imprinting is considered to be a particular type of epigenetic modification in which changes occur in the transcriptional control of genes.

Two lines of evidence have been presented by Traupe *et al.*[14] which suggest that genomic imprinting of a major gene occurs in psoriasis. Firstly, the birth weight of children from psoriatics is influenced by the sex of the psoriatic parent (children from fathers with psoriasis are significantly heavier than children from psoriatic mothers), and secondly, the disease manifestation or penetrance depends in part upon the sex of the psoriatic parent. The latter was demonstrated by the re-analysis of the Faroe Island pedigrees[6] which showed that fathers with psoriasis more often have affected children than mothers with psoriasis. This was also true for offspring of male "gene carriers" — clinically healthy persons who have a first- or second-degree relative with psoriasis and therefore presumably carry a major gene for psoriasis in their family.

Further evidence for a parental sex effect with more probands having an affected father than an affected mother has recently been reported.[15] Furthermore, genetic anticipation (increase in disease severity or decrease in age at onset in successive generations) was also apparent and most marked if the disease was inherited from the father.[15]

1.2.4 *HLA Associations*

In common with most autoimmune diseases, psoriasis is associated with several HLA antigens. They include the Class I antigens, HLA-B13, -B17, -B37, -B57, -Cw6 and -Cw7, and the Class II antigens HLA-DR7 and HLA-DR4.[16-18] The Cw6 allele, which is in linkage disequilibrium with B13, B17 and B37, shows the strongest association in psoriasis and correlates with early onset and positive family history

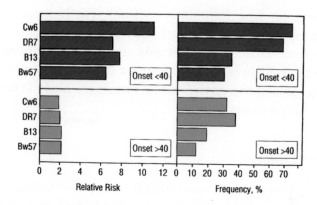

Fig. 1.3. Increased relative risk of HLA Cw6 and HLA-DR7 in juvenile onset psoriasis. (Sources: Reprinted from Elder *et al.*, Arch Dermatol **130** (1994), 216–224; *Psoriasis* Marcel Dekker, New York, pp. 15–21, 1990, with permission from the American Medical Association, Chicago, USA.)

(type I psoriasis)[19] (Fig. 1.3). Furthermore, the HLA Class II extended haplotype DRB1*0701/2, DQA1*0201, DQB1*0303 has been found exclusively in type I psoriasis.[20]

The analysis of polymerase chain reaction (PCR)-amplified HLA-C gene segments in Japanese psoriasis patients revealed a strong association between psoriasis and alanine at position 73 on the α1 domain helix that forms one side of the putative antigen-binding cleft of HLA-C molecules.[21] Although the unique substitution of [73]Ala for [73]Thr is common to CW6 and CW7, HLA-CW4 which is not associated with psoriasis also shared this substitution, whilst CW11, which is strongly associated in Japanese patients, did not. Furthermore, in a similar study of psoriasis patients of white European extraction, no association between the [73]Ala coding nucleotide sequence and psoriasis was detected[22] raising doubts as to the significance of the Japanese findings.

The observation that the HLA alleles associated with psoriasis are in linkage disequilibrium suggests that susceptibility to psoriasis involves a gene(s) close to, but separate from HLA Class I genes on chromosome 6p (see following section). Furthermore, the small proportion (approximately 10%) of HLA-predisposed individuals who actually go on to develop psoriasis implies that inheritance of a particular HLA allele is not sufficient for development of the disease. In addition, gene(s) and enviromental factors are likely to be necessary for triggering psoriasis.

1.2.5 *Gene Linkage*

Since 1994, three main susceptibility loci for familial psoriasis have been reported on chromosomes 17q,[23] 4q[24] and 6p.[25,26] These studies involved genome-wide linkage analysis with polymorphic microsatellite markers on multiplex families and/or affected sibling pairs. Lod score analysis was used to determine the linkage. "Lod" represents the logarithm of odds ratio and refers to the likelihood that a particular pattern of inheritance of a genetic marker would be observed if the marker is close to the disease gene (linked), relative to that marker being located far away (unlinked). A lod score of ≥ 3.0 is taken as indicative of linkage. Since the mode of inheritance is unknown, non-parametric methods of data analysis which identify regions of excess allele sharing were also used. These studies have demonstrated genetic heterogeneity. Thus, none of the families with linkage to chromosome 17q showed any association with Cw6.[23] However, in the second study, only one of seven predominately Irish families showed linkage to chromosome 17q, whilst four out of six families showed cosegregation of psoriasis with a chromosome 4q haplotype.[24] Furthermore, the chromosome 4q linkage site has not been confirmed in three further studies in which the patients were not of Irish descent[15,25,26] suggesting a founder effect in the Irish population.

In contrast, the susceptibility locus on chromosome 6, located in the MHC cluster region p21.3, has been independently confirmed by three groups.[15,25,26] Linkage analysis of HLA markers in familial psoriasis suggest that this major determinant resides within the region

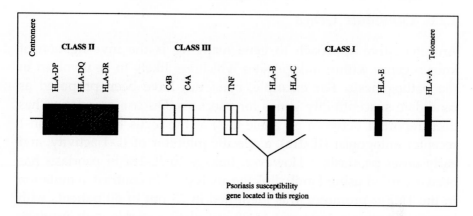

Fig. 1.4. Region of human chromosome 6p21.3 containing psoriasis susceptibility gene.

extending from just telomeric to the tumor necrosis factor-β (TNFB) gene to approximately 100 kb telomeric to HLA-C (Fig. 1.4).[27]

In addition to the main loci mentioned above, further linkage sites have been described on chromosomes 1, 2, 8, 16q and 20p.[25,26,28] Interestingly, the region on chromosome 16q overlaps with a recently identified susceptibility locus for Crohn's disease,[26] which could explain the strong concomitance of psoriasis and Crohn's disease.[29] Furthermore, a linkage site on chromosome 4q has been identified in a subset of mixed families, containing one member with Crohn's disease and another with ulcerative colitis, especially among Ashkenazim.[30] Whether this is located near the 4q linkage site in psoriatic families has yet to be determined.

Once gene linkage sites have been localized, the next step is the identification of the affected gene(s). Powerful and sensitive techniques such as linkage disequilibrium mapping can be used to significantly reduce the size of the linked region to enable this to be achieved. Despite the complexities of the inheritance of psoriasis, identification of the genes that determine susceptibility to psoriasis is now feasible and likely to be made in the near, rather than distant, future.

1.2.6. *Candidate Genes*

An alternative approach to gene mapping is the investigation of known genes within linkage sites which are likely to be involved in the pathogenesis. For example, cytokines have been proposed as candidate susceptibility genes for psoriasis. Disease association has been reported between an allele (A2) at the locus for Interleukin-1 receptor antagonist (IL-1ra), a specific inhibitor of IL-1 activity, and early onset psoriasis.[31] However, linkage to IL-1ra in psoriasis has been excluded using family linkage analysis.[32] In contrast, a mutation in the TNF-α promotor was identified in 23 out of 60 patients with juvenile onset psoriasis and in 20 out of 62 patients with psoriatic arthritis compared with 7 out of 99 Caucasian controls.[33] There was also a marked increase of homozygotes for this mutation in the psoriatic group. The TNF-α gene is located on chromosome 6p21.3 within the Class III region of the MHC between HLA-B and HLA-DR (Fig. 1.4). The functional consequences of this polymorphism in affected individuals are unknown, but altered TNF-α secretion is likely. The role of TNF-α in psoriasis is discussed in Sec. 6.1.8.

Polymorphisms of the IFN-γ and IL-10 genes associated with different levels of cytokine production have also been studied in patients with psoriasis.[34] There was no detection of any significant difference in the genotypes expressed by psoriatic patients compared to controls or between early and late onset psoriasis. This suggested that the predominance of TH_1 cytokines in psoriatic skin lesions could not be explained on the basis of altered gene expression of IFN-γ and IL-10.

Another candidate gene investigated, the S gene, was recently identified in the HLA Class I region located 160 kb telomeric of HLA-C which encodes a keratin-like protein and is expressed specifically in the granular layer of the epidermis.[35] Two diallelic polymorphic sites in exon 1, and seven dialleleic polymorphic sites in exon 2, three of which result in amino acid exchanges, have been identified. No significant differences in dimorphic distributions between psoriatic patients and healthy controls were detected in one study,[36] but more recently an association between psoriasis and the S gene polymorphism at position 1243 was detected particularly in patients with early onset disease.[37]

1.3 Environmental Factors

Various environmental factors can initiate or exacerbate the disease, although their effects may vary between individuals presumably due to modifying factors (Table 1.1).

Upper respiratory tract infection by β-haemolytic, group A streptococci has long been recognised as a trigger for guttate psoriasis. This infection can also exacerbate the chronic form of the disease.[38] More recently, the appearance and/or marked worsening of psoriasis in patients infected with the HIV virus has been reported.[39] It is not clear whether the virus itself, or one or more of the associated opportunistic bacterial infections is responsible for activation of the disease in these patients. Local infection with *S. aureus* and *C. albicans* has also been associated with the exacerbation of psoriasis.[40]

Table 1.1   Enviromental factors that provoke or exacerbate psoriasis

Factor	Reported Association
Infection	Steptococcus pyogenes
	HIV (opportunistic infections)
	Staphylococcus aureus
	Candida albicans
	Pityrosporum (Malassesia furfur)
	Retroviruses
Trauma	Physical, chemical, surgical (Koebner reaction)
Endocrine factors	Pregnancy, oestrogen therapy, stress
Drugs	Lithium, anti-malarials, β-blockers,
	Withdrawal of systemic corticosteroids
Metabolic factors	Hypocalcaemia
Alcohol	Heavy consumption

Furthermore, both *retroviruses* and *Pityrosporum* yeasts have been proposed as possible triggers.[41,42]

Development of psoriasis at the site of injury on uninvolved skin — the Koebner phenomenon — has been well documented in response to many types of trauma such as scratches, bites and tattoos. Damage to the epidermis is necessary to produce a reaction.[43] In a given patient, if the response is positive at one site, it will also be positive at other sites at the same point in time. However, a positive response will only be observed in a proportion (approximately 25%) of a randomly selected group of patients at any given time. The clearing of existing psoriasis following an injury has also been observed and referred to as the "reverse Koebner".[44] This is also an all-or-none phenomenon, and the Koebner and reverse Koebner are mutually exclusive. These observations suggest the presence of systemic factors which modulate the expression of the disease. The finding that serum from patients recovering from active psoriasis inhibits the Koebner reaction lends support to this idea.[45]

Although psoriasis may worsen during pregnancy, it is more likely to improve or remain unchanged. Stress is often associated with the exacerbation of psoriasis and this could be explained by the effects on the immune system via stress-induced alterations in hormone levels. Various drugs can also induce psoriasis especially the administration of lithium, β-blockers such as practolol, and anti-malarials, and the withdrawal of systemically administered corticosteroids. Other factors include hypocalcaemia and heavy consumption of alcohol.

1.4 Histological Features

The major histological features of a psoriatic plaque are a hyperproliferative epidermal layer together with a mononuclear cellular infiltrate surrounding dilated and tortuous capillaries in the papillary dermis (Fig. 1.5).

The epidermis is characterised by a parakeratotic stratum corneum containing aggregates of neutrophils (Munro abscesses), absence of a

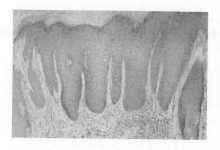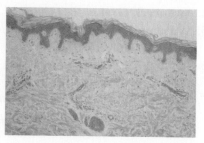

Fig. 1.5. Histology of a psoriatic plaque (*left*) compared to normal skin (*right*).

granular layer, thinning of the suprapapillary plate, and regular elongation of the rete ridges with clubbing. These features demonstrate a large increase in the numbers of epidermal cells (by a factor of 4 as compared to normal skin) together with abnormal keratinization. However, the increase in the rate of production of epidermal cells in a psoriatic lesion is probably not the result of an altered cell cycle time, as previously believed. Recent evidence suggests that hyperproliferation is due to the activation of, but not an increase in, the normally quiescent basal keratinocyte cell population which includes the stem cells. This is accompanied by accelerated maturation and differentiation.[46]

However, these epidermal changes are secondary to the appearance of a perivascular mononuclear cell infiltrate, as well as. dilation and tortuosity of the blood vessels in the dermal papillae which are the earliest histological changes in the formation of a psoriatic lesion.[47] The majority of mononuclear cells in the infiltrate of both early and fully developed psoriatic lesions are T lymphocytes, macrophages and dendritic cells, with very few B lymphocytes or neutrophils.

References

1. Leczinsky C.G. *Acta Dermatol.Venereol. (Stockh)* **28** (1948), 483–487.
2. Scarpa R. *et al. Br.J.Rheumatol.* **23** (1984), 246–250.
3. Yates V.M., Watkinson G., Kelman A. *Br.J.Dermatol.* **106** (1982), 323–330.

4. Swanbeck G. *et al. Br.J.Dermatol.* **133** (1995), 768–773.
5. Williams R.C., McKenzie A.W., Roger J.H., Joysey V.C. *Br.J.Dermatol.* **95** (1976), 163–167.
6. Lomholt G. *Psoriasis: Prevalence, Spontaneous Course and Genetics.* G.E.C. Gad, Copenhagen (1963).
7. Hellgren I. *Psoriasis: The Prevalence in Sex, Age and Occupational Groups in Total Populations in Sweden: Morphology, Inheritance and Association With Other Skin and Rheumatic Diseases.* Almqvist & Wiksell, Stockholm (1967).
8. Elder J.T. *et al. Arch.Dermatol.* **130** (1994), 216–224.
9. Brandrup F. *et al. Acta Dermatol.* **62** (1982), 229–236.
10. Farber E.M., Nall I., Watson W. *Arch.Dermatol.* **109** (1974), 207–211.
11. Abele D.C., Dobson R.L., Graham J.B., Hill C. *Arch.Dermatol.* **88** (1963), 89–99.
12. Swanbeck G., Inerot A., Martinsson T., Wahlstrom J. *Br.J.Dermatol.* **131** (1994), 32–39.
13. Watson W., Cann H.M., Farber E.M., Nall M.L. *Arch.Dermatol.* **105** (1972), 197–207.
14. Traupe H. *et al. Am.J.Med.Genet.* **42** (1992), 649–654.
15. Burden A.D. *et al. J.Invest.Dermatol.* **110** (1998), 958–960.
16. Svejgaard A. *et al. Br.J.Dermatol.* **91** (1974), 145–153.
17. Tiilikainen A. *et al. Br.J.Dermatol.* **102** (1980), 179–184.
18. Tiwari J.L. *et al. Br.J.Dermatol.* **106** (1982), 227–230.
19. Henseler T. and Christophers E. *J.Am.Acad.Dermatol.* **13** (1985), 450–456.
20. Schmitt-Egenolf M. *et al. J.Invest.Dermatol.* **100** (1993), 749–752.
21. Asahina A. *et al. J.Invest.Dermatol.* **97** (1991), 254–258.
22. Chew E. *et al. Br.J.Dermatol.* **135** (1996), 825 (Abstract).
23. Tomfohrde T. *et al. Science* **264** (1994), 1141–1145.
24. Matthews D. *et al. Nature Genetics* **14** (1996), 231–233.
25. Trembath R.C. *et al. Hum.Mol.Genet.* **6** (1997), 813–820.
26. Nair R.P. *et al. Hum.Mol.Genet.* **6** (1997), 1349–1356.
27. Jenisch S. *et al. Am.J.Hum.Genet.* **63** (1998), 191–199.
28. Capon F. *et al. J.Invest.Dermatol.* **112** (1999), 32–35.
29. Lee F.I., Bellary S.V., Francis C. *Am.J.Gastroenterol.* **85** (1990), 962–963.
30. Cho J.H. *et al. Proc.Natl.Acad.Sci. (USA)* **95** (1998), 7502–7507.
31. Tarlow J.K. *et al. Br.J.Dermatol.* **136** (1997), 147–148.
32. Rosbotham J.L., Barker J.N.W.N., Trembath R.C. *J.Invest.Dermatol.* **104** (1995), 306 (Letter).

33. Hohler T. *et al.* *J.Invest.Dermatol.* **109** (1997), 562–565.
34. Craven N.M. *et al.* *Br.J.Dermatol.* **139, Suppl.** 51 (1998), 26.
35. Zhou Y. and Chaplin D.D. *Proc.Natl.Acad.Sci. (USA)* **90** (1993), 9470–9474.
36. Ishihara M. *et al.* *Tissue Antigens* **48** (1996), 182–186.
37. Ahnini T. *et al.* *Hum.Mol.Genet.* **8** (1999), 1135–1140.
38. Cohen-Tervaert W.C. and Esseveld H. *Dermatologica* **140** (1970), 282–290.
39. Duvic M. *et al.* *Arch.Dermatol.* **123** (1987), 1622–1632.
40. Leung D.Y.M., Walsh P., Storno R., Norris D.A. *J.Invest.Dermatol.* **100** (1993), 225–228.
41. Iversen O.J., Nissen-Meyjer J., Dalen A.B. *Acta Pathol.Microbiol.Immunol. (Scand)* **91** (1983), 413–417.
42. Rosenberg E.W. and Belew P.W. *Arch.Dermatol.* **118** (1982), 370–371.
43. Pedace J., Muller A., Winkelmann R.K. *Acta Dermatol.Venereol. (Stockh)* **49** (1969), 390–400.
44. Eyre R.W. and Krueger G.G. *Br.J.Dermatol.* **106** (1982), 153–159.
45. Stankler L. *Br.J.Dermatol.* **91, Suppl.** 10 (1974), 15.
46. Bata-Csorgo Z., Hammerberg C., Vorhees J.J., Cooper K.D. *J.Exp.Med.* **178** (1993), 1271–1281.
47. Ragaz A. and Ackerman A.B. *Am.J.Dermatopathol.* **1** (1979), 199–214.

CHAPTER 2

Skin Immune System in Psoriasis

2.1 Skin Immune System (SIS)

Normal human skin is no longer regarded merely as a protective covering for the body, but as a complex immunological unit. In 1978, Streilin[1] coined the term "skin-associated lymphoid tissues" (SALT) to describe the following immunocompetent cells in the epidermis:

1. Epidermotropic recirculating T lymphocyte subpopulations (homing T lymphocytes);
2. Langerhans cells with antigen-presenting capabilities;
3. Keratinocytes producing epidermal thymocyte-activating factor, later identified as Interleukin-1;
4. Skin-draining peripheral lymph nodes which include vascular high endothelial cells with the capacity to capture lymphocytes passing through the blood.

However, in addition to these epidermal cells, a number of other immunologically active cells are present in the (epi)dermal layers of the skin such as mast cells, tissue macrophages, neutrophilic granulocytes, indeterminate cells, veiled cells, vascular endothelial cells, and afferent lymphatic endothelium beginning in the dermis. Subsequently, Bos and Kapsenberg proposed the term "Skin Immune System" (SIS) to encompass these cell types together with those of SALT, but excluding skin-draining lymph nodes (Fig. 2.1).[2]

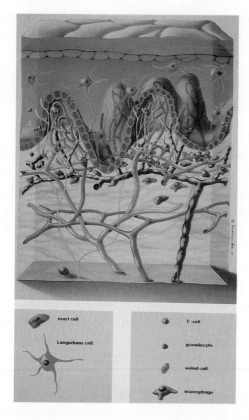

Fig. 2.1. Schematic representation of the cellular constituents of the skin immune system (SIS). (Source: Bos J.D. *Skin Immune System* (1990), with permission from CRC Press Inc., Boca Raton, Florida, USA.)

Immunocompetent cells in the skin can be resident, recruited and/or recirculating. Eosinophils, for example, are recruited to the skin only in certain pathological states, unlike T lymphocytes which are resident in small numbers and recirculate between the skin and the skin-draining lymph nodes.

In addition to the cellular constituents of the SIS, a variety of inflammatory and immune mediators are also present in normal skin. These may be produced *in situ* or enter the skin via the circulation and include anti-microbial peptides, complement components, immunoglobulins, cytokines, fibrinolysins, eicosanoids and neuropeptides.

2.2 T Cell Subpopulations: Normal Skin

Prior to 1980, T lymphocytes in peripheral blood and tissues (including psoriatic skin) were studied using enzyme cytochemical methods, sheep red blood cell rosetting or haemadsorption, or by immuno-staining with polyclonal anti-T cell antisera. With the advent of monoclonal antibody hybridoma technology, introduced by Kohler and Milstein in 1975, it became possible, for the first time, to identify subpopulations of immune cells using highly specific probes for surface markers.

T lymphocytes which have matured in the thymus from bone-marrow-derived precursors can be subdivided into two functionally distinct subpopulations based on the expression of CD4 or CD8 molecules on the cell surface. CD4+ T cells interact with MHC Class II molecules on the surface of antigen-presenting cells, such as dendritic cells, B cells and macrophages, in the groove of which antigenic peptides are bound. They function as "helper" T cells assisting B cells to produce immunoglobulins and inducing the maturation of cytotoxic T cells via the production of cytokines. CD8+ T cells, on the other hand, interact in an antigen-specific manner with MHC Class I products expressed on the surface of all nucleated cells. They function as either cytotoxic T cells or as suppressors of antigen-specific B and T cell responses. Subsequent to activation, molecules such as the Interleukin-2 receptor (IL-2R) and MHC Class II HLA-DR, which are absent on resting T cells, are upregulated on the surface of both CD4+ and CD8+ T cells.

Although quantification of intraepidermal T lymphocytes in earlier studies gave inconsistent results, several subsequent studies have confirmed the presence of a small numbers of T cells in normal skin.[3-5] Intraepidermal T cells, which account for less than 2% of the total number of skin lymphocytes, are predominately CD8[+3,4] and express the more common T cell receptor consisting of a heterodimer of α and β chains (TCR$\alpha\beta$).[4] The majority of T cells in normal skin are clustered in 1–3 rows around post-capillary venules of the papillary vascular plexus or adjacent to cutaneous appendages. In contrast to circulating T cells, most of the perivascular T cells express HLA-DR and IL-2R molecules. Moreover, they consist of approximately equal numbers of CD4[+], 4B4[+] memory (previously known as helper-inducer) and CD8[+] T cell subsets, whilst CD4[+] and CD45RA[+] (2H4[+]) naive T cells, formerly described as suppressor-inducer T cells, are relatively rare. This differs markedly from peripheral blood in which approximately 50% of circulating CD4[+] T cells are CD45RA[+].

These observations suggest that the majority of CD4[+] T cells comprising the perivascular infiltrate in normal skin have previously encountered antigen in the context of MHC Class II antigen. It is not known whether these T cells enter the skin in an activated state or are activated *in situ*. The latter appears more likely because of the spatial relationship to antigen-presenting cells such as dermal dendritic and endothelial cells (as discussed in the following section) and the chronic exposure of the skin to exogenous antigens.

2.3 T Cell Subpopulations: Psoriatic Skin

The clinically uninvolved skin of patients with psoriasis, although histologically normal, shows an increase in both T cell infiltration and epidermal proliferation.[6] Small numbers of CD8[+] T cells are more frequently present in the basal epidermis of uninvolved psoriatic compared to normal skin, whilst in the dermis there is a marked increase in CD4[+] and, to a lesser extent, CD8[+] T cells.[3] Furthermore, activated dermal CD4[+] T cells are commonly present whilst HLA-DR expression by CD8[+] T cells is less frequently observed.[3]

The transition from uninvolved to lesional skin is associated with the epidermal influx and activation of CD4[+] T cells as observed in very early lesions (less than 2 mm in diameter, less than 1 week old) of guttate psoriasis.[3] These CD4[+] T cells are seen in the basal epidermal layer in close proximity to HLA-DR[+] epidermal dendritic cells (Fig. 2.2). In contrast, the appearance of a clinical lesion is not accompanied by detectable changes in the numbers of T cells in the dermis.[3]

In the early lesion, the ratio of epidermal CD4[+] : CD8[+] T cells is approximately 1.0. However, this decreases to approximately 0.5 in late lesions (more than 1 cm in diameter, 3–8 weeks old, some of which are fading) due to an influx of CD8[+] T cells.[3,7] A proportion of the CD8[+] T cells expresses HLA-DR antigen whilst, in contrast to early lesions, CD4[+] T cells are not activated although their numbers are similar to that of the early lesions. In these late lesions, both CD4[+] T cells, and more frequently CD8[+] T cells, are seen in close proximity to HLA-DR[+] dendritic cells (Fig. 2.3). These findings were supported by a longitudinal study on a single patient with guttate psoriasis who was sequentially biopsied over a 4–15 week period after the onset of lesions during which active lesions gradually began to fade spontaneously. The number of CD4[+] T cells declined progressively accompanied by a corresponding increase in CD8[+] T cells (Fig. 2.4).

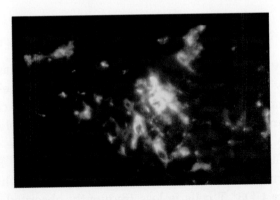

Fig. 2.2. Double immunostaining of an early guttate lesion with Leu 3a (CD4[+] T cells, red) and anti-HLA-DR (dendritic cells, green) antibodies. (Source: Baker B.S. *et al. Clin.Exp.Immunol.* **61** (1985), 526–534, with permission from Blackwell Science Ltd, Oxford, UK.)

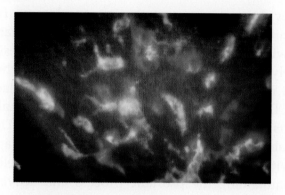

Fig. 2.3. Double immunostaining of a late guttate lesion with Leu 2a (CD8⁺ T cells, red) and anti-HLA-DR (dendritic cells, green) antibodies.

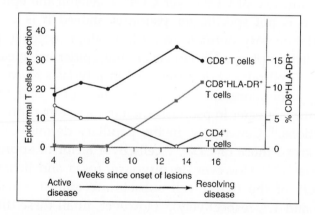

Fig. 2.4. Longitudinal study of epidermal T cells in a patient with guttate psoriasis. (Source: Valdimarsson H. *et al. Immunol.Today* **16** (1995), 145–149, with permission from Elsevier Science, Oxford, UK.)

Furthermore, at 12 weeks, a significant number of HLA-DR⁺ CD8⁺ T cells appeared, coinciding with resolution of the lesions.

Thus, the clinical activity of psoriasis appears to be dependent upon the interaction of CD4⁺ and CD8⁺ T cells with antigen-presenting cells in the epidermis.

Further evidence to support this proposal came from similar immunostaining studies of stable chronic plaque psoriatic lesions.[8,9] In common with resolving guttate lesions, the chronic lesions showed approximately twice as many CD8+ as CD4+ T cells in the epidermis. However, in contrast to the resolving lesions which lack activated epidermal CD4+ T cells, equal numbers of epidermal CD4+ and CD8+ T cells in persistent plaques express HLA-DR antigen.[8] Thus, the stability of chronic plaque psoriatic lesions appears to be associated with a balance between activated CD4+ T cells capable of initiating/maintaining the psoriatic process and activated CD8+ T cells potentially able to switch it off. Alternatively, it is possible that these CD8+ T cells may have an effector role. This is discussed in Sec. 8.4.

A predominance of CD8+ over CD4+ T cells in the epidermis of lesional skin is not specific for psoriasis, indeed it is common to various inflammatory dermatoses such as atopic eczema, pityriasis rosea and lichen planus.[9,10] However, the epidermal mean CD4+/ mean CD8+ T cell ratio varies from 0.04 in pityriasis rosea to 0.48 in psoriasis.[9] Furthermore, the absolute numbers of T cells infiltrating the epidermis is greater in psoriasis than in these other inflammatory skin conditions.[10] Conversely, in the papillary dermis, CD4+ T cell numbers exceed those of CD8+ T cells by a factor of approximately 2.6 in psoriasis.[9,11] However, in pityriasis rosea and lichen planus, the numbers of the two T cell subsets are almost equal (CD4+/ CD8+ = 1.4 and 1.1, respectively).[9] However, in all these diseases, as in normal skin discussed above, the CD4+ T cells in both epidermis and dermis are almost exclusively (more than 95%) of the 4B4+, 2H4-, Cdw29+ memory T cell subpopulation whereas 4B4-, 2H4+, CD45RA+ naive T cells are extremely uncommon in lesional epidermis.

This predominance of the memory T cell subpopulation indicates that most CD4+ T cells in both normal and diseased human skin are already primed to their specific antigenic determinant in the context of MHC Class II. However, disease-specific patterns of T cell subset infiltration exist in different inflammatory skin dermatoses. This may be relevant to the specific immunopathogenic mechanisms involved in each case.

2.4 Antigen-Presenting Cells: Normal Skin

Antigen-presenting cells (APC) in normal skin include dendritic cells (epidermal Langerhans and dermal dendritic), indeterminate cells and dermal macrophages.

2.4.1 *Epidermal Dendritic Cells*

Dendritic cells (DC) were originally described by Steinman and Cohen[12] as a novel cell type in murine spleen suspensions. Since then, an understanding of the DC lineage has emerged.[13] Thus DC progenitors originating in the bone marrow enter the blood and seed non-lymphoid tissues such as the skin, gut, genito-urinary tract and lung epithelia where they develop into so called "immature" DCs capable of antigen uptake and processing, MHC production and the formation of foreign peptide-MHC complexes. Cytokines and other factors then induce their maturation and migration out of non-lymphoid tissues into the blood and/or afferent lymph (veiled cells). DCs migrating into secondary lymphoid tissues acquire the ability to initiate primary T cell immune reactions via upregulation of costimulatory molecule expression and synthesis of cytokines such as IL-12 (mature DCs).

Langerhans cells (LCs), which are used as a prototype for studies of DCs, reside in the suprabasal layer of the epidermis forming a regular network with their dendrites, and were originally detected by staining for ATPase activity. The LC cell surface expresses an array of molecules including MHC Class II subtypes, HLA-DR, -DP and -DQ which are constitutively expressed (Fig. 2.5), and InterCellular Adhesion Molecule-1 and -3 (ICAM-1,3) and Lymphocyte Functional Antigen-3 (LFA-3) which, together with MHC Class II molecules, are involved in antigen presentation to T cells. The latter

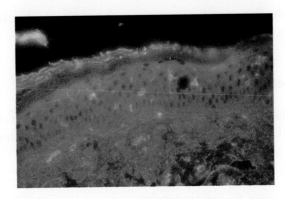

Fig. 2.5. Langerhans cells in normal epidermis stained for HLA-DR antigen.

group of molecules is detected on freshly isolated cells together with Fc receptor (FcR) and Complement 3bi receptor (C3biR).

In common with monocytes and macrophages, low levels of CD4 glycoprotein, which was originally thought to be exclusively expressed by subpopulations of T cells are present on the LC surface. In addition, LCs express CD1, a non-polymorphic MHC Class I-like molecule encoded for by genes which, unlike those coding for MHC molecules, do not map to chromosome 6.[14] The human CD1 locus contains five genes — the protein products of three of these genes CD1a, b and c have been identified as β_2-microglobulin-associated cell surface glycoproteins on immature thymocytes. CD1a is also expressed by epidermal LCs[15] and CD1c by dermal DCs[16] and a subpopulation of B cells. The function of CD1 on LCs is presently unknown but may, in common with MHC molecules, bind antigen prior to internalisation.

Within their cytoplasm, LCs characteristically contain unique rod-like organelles called Birbeck granules — named after the person who first described them,[17] — which can be found in association with small vesicles forming racket-like structures. The precise function of these organelles is still unknown, but it is likely that they result from sandwiching of the plasma membrane initiated by cross-linking of cell surface structures, including perhaps CD1a.

Thus freshly isolated LCs are capable of pinocytosis and processing of soluble antigens targeted by the cells' membrane molecules, which are subsequently expressed as peptide-MHC complexes at the cell surface. However, they are unable to initiate primary *in vitro* immune responses. During culture in the presence of Granulocyte Macrophage-Colony Stimulating Factor (GM-CSF), FcR and CD1a are down-regulated together with the capacity to process soluble antigens, but molecules necessary for antigen presentation (HLA Class II, ICAM-1, LFA-3) are preserved. In addition, cultured human LCs acquire expression of RFD-1, a characteristic MHC Class II marker of IDC,[18] interdigitating cells found in the T cell compartments of lymphoid tissues. These cultured cells are therefore equivalent to the mature DCs that migrate via the dermal lymph to skin-associated lymph nodes where they initiate primary T cell immune responses.

2.4.2 *Dermal Dendritic Cells (DDC)*

DCs are also present around the vessels of the papillary dermis of normal skin (DDC) and express Factor XIIIa, an intracellular form of fibrin stabilizing factor,[19] and either CD1a or RFD1. Cultured DDC exhibit high surface expression of B7 (which binds to CD28 on T cells and delivers a potent costimulatory signal), HLA-DR, and the adhesion molecule CD11a (LFA-1).[20] Further analysis of the subtypes of B7 revealed that B7-2 (CD86) is expressed at higher levels than B7-1 (CD80) in contrast to cultured monocytes that express low and equivalent levels of B7-1 and B7-2.[21]

2.4.3 *Indeterminate Cells*

Indeterminate cells have a morphology resembling LCs but lack the LC-characteristic Birbeck organelles. They appear to be intermediate between LCs and their precursors and may be regarded as migrating cells being observed in both epidermis and dermis. However, it is possible that these cells do not in fact exist as a separate cell type but result from inadequate sectioning which fails to reveal the presence of the Birbeck granules.

2.4.4 *Macrophages*

In normal skin, abundant macrophages are found in the superficial dermis adjacent to small vessels, and scattered in the reticular dermis. Macrophages are bone-marrow-derived cells which are regarded as distinct from DCs but which are probably derived from a common precursor. The environment in which the cells differentiate probably determines which cell type is produced. Macrophages are highly phagocytic and act as scavengers of cellular debris and of organisms which breach the epidermal barrier. They probably also act as antigen-presenting cells although this has not yet been demonstrated *in situ* in skin.

2.5 Antigen-Presenting Cells: Psoriatic Skin

2.5.1 *Epidermal Dendritic Cells*

There have been conflicting reports concerning the numbers of LCs in psoriatic epidermis. Two reports employing ATPase staining, and single staining with monoclonal anti-HLA-DR or anti-CD1 antibodies, respectively[7,22] suggested that epidermal LC numbers were decreased but actual numbers of cells were not presented. Both studies also noted that the LCs had shorter dendritic processes than those of the cells in normal skin. In contrast, quantitation of LC numbers in the epidermis of chronic plaque lesions using double-immunostaining for HLA-DR and CD1a antigens, revealed a marked increase in the total number of epidermal DCs compared to both uninvolved psoriatic and normal skin and, to a lesser extent, in uninvolved compared to normal skin.[8] Furthermore, 82% of LCs in lesional epidermis expressed HLA-DR compared to only 50% in normal and uninvolved psoriatic epidermis (Table 2.1).

Table 2.1 Subpopulations of epidermal dendritic cells in lesional, uninvolved psoriatic and normal skin. (Source: Baker B.S. *et al. Clin.Exp.Immunol.* **61** (1985), 526–534, with permission from Blackwell Science Ltd, Oxford, UK.)

Skin	DR+CD1+		DR+CD1−		DR−CD1+		Total Dendritic Cells
	No./50HPF	%	No./50HPF	%	No./50HPF	%	
Normal (n = 13)	227 ± 31 (94–470)	50 ± 4.0	np	np	209 ± 12 (124–288)	50 ± 4.0	437 ± 30 (304–621)
Uninvolved Psoriatic (n = 18)	288 ± 29 (125–611)	54 ± 3.1	np	np	256 ± 22 (137 ± 473)	46 ± 3.1	547 ± 38† (294–922)
Lesional Psoriatic (n = 18)	525 ± 44* (134–892)	66 ± 2.8	128 ± 20 (32–330)	18 ± 2.9	122 ± 15* (19–256)	16 ± 1.6	775 ± 49* (359–1,193)

Results expressed as means ± standard error, ranges in brackets. np = None present. n = Number of biopsies examined.
*Lesional *vs* normal/uninvolved psoriatic, $p < 0.001$.
†Uninvolved psoriatic *vs* normal, $p < 0.05$.

Interestingly, the DR+ LCs in lesional epidermis included a subpopulation of cells (18%) which did not appear to express the CD1a epitope but contained Birbeck granules (Fig. 2.6). Such DR+ CD1a− cells were rarely seen in the epidermis of normal controls or in uninvolved epidermis from psoriatic patients.

However, this cell type is not unique to psoriasis, but is found in other benign inflammatory skin diseases such as endogenous eczema, pityriasis rosea and lichen planus.[23] Furthermore, *non-Langerhans* DR+ CD1a− cells expressing Hle1 antigen found on all bone-marrow-derived leukocytes, have also been demonstrated in lesional psoriatic epidermis.[24] These cells, which include monocytes and RFD1+ cells, showed enhanced capacity to activate and induce proliferation of T lymphocytes and differ from, but are analogous to, DR+ CD1a− epidermal cells that appear following UV exposure of the skin.[25]

In addition to increased numbers, the distribution of LCs in psoriatic epidermis is altered with marked clumping in the upper

(a)

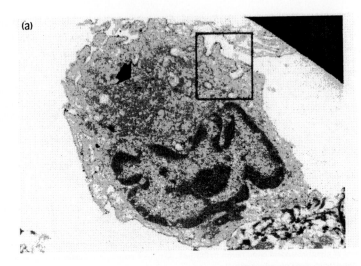

Fig. 2.6(a). A Langerhans cell observed in the epidermal sheet from a psoriatic lesion showing labelling with large (CD1) and small (HLA-DR) gold granules. Arrow indicates Birbeck granules in the cytoplasm. (Source: Figs. 2.6 a–d. Reprinted from Baker B.S. *et al. Acta Dermatol.Venereol.* **68** (1988), 209–217, with permission from Scandinavian University Press, Oslo, Norway.)

(b)

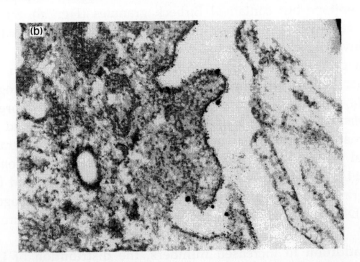

Fig. 2.6(b). Higher magnification of the boxed area in (a) showing gold granules in close apposition with the cell membrane.

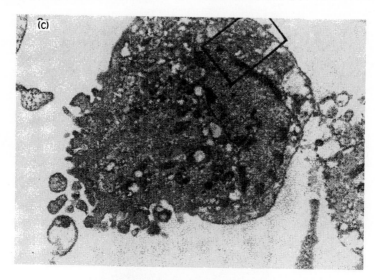

Fig. 2.6(c). A Langerhans cell observed in the epidermal sheet from a psoriatic lesion showing heavy labelling with small gold granules (HLA-DR antigen) and very few large gold granules (CD1 antigen).

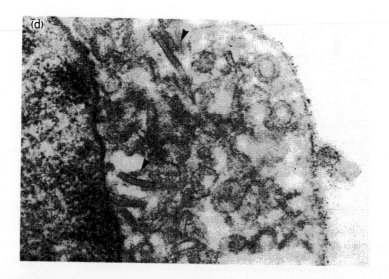

Fig. 2.6(d). Higher magnification of the boxed area in (c) showing Birbeck granules (arrowheads).

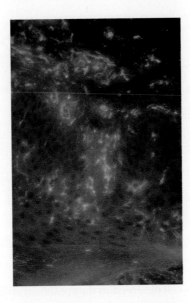

Fig. 2.7. Marked clumping of Langerhans cells stained for HLA-DR antigen in the epidermis of a psoriatic lesion.

epidermal layers and scattered cells in the rete ridges (Fig. 2.7).[3,7,8] This finding appears to be characteristic for psoriasis and is not observed in other inflammatory dermatoses.

2.5.2 *Dermal Dendritic Cells (DDC)*

Dermal dendritic cells (DDC) are increased in psoriatic lesions and both CD1a[+] and RFD1[+] interdigitating dendritic cells are observed in close conjunction with T cells in cellular infiltrates of the papillary dermis.[26] This pattern is also observed in atopic dermatitis, whereas in pityriasis rosea a higher percentage of CD1a[+] LCs and lower numbers of RFD1[+] interdigitating dendritic cells are present.[26] In other dermatoses such as allergic contact dermatitis, lichen planus and lupus erythematosus, both dendritic cell subsets are poorly represented.[26]

Thus, in psoriasis (and atopic dermatitis), antigen presentation by DDC to T cells appears to be an important feature of the pathogenesis.

2.6 Endothelial Cells

Histological studies have shown that the earliest changes in psoriatic skin occur in the dermal microvasculature.[27] Microvessels in the papillary dermis are elongated, dilated and hyperpermeable, and undergo angiogenesis and high endothelial venule (HEV) formation.

Angiogenesis refers to the formation of new capillary blood vessels from the existing microvascular bed, and is a highly regulated process resulting from a balance between inducers, for example, acidic and basic fibroblast growth factors (FGF), transforming growth factor-α (TGF-α) and tumour necrosis factor-α (TNF-α), and inhibitors such as platelet factor-4 and thrombospondin. Normally inhibitors of angiogenesis maintain the capillary endothelium in a quiescent state.[28] However, in psoriatic lesions, angiogenesis is stimulated compared to that of normal skin, as suggested by increased ^{3}H-thymidine labelling of dermal endothelial cells[29] and increased number and mass of capillary blood vessels.[30] There is also an increase of the enzyme capillary alkaline phosphatase, a marker of new dermal capillaries, in developing psoriatic plaques.[31]

In vitro, it was demonstrated that both peripheral blood mononuclear cells and sera from patients with active psoriasis could induce new blood vessel formation,[32] but experiments testing the angiogenic activity of psoriatic epidermis *in vivo* gave conflicting results. These observations could be explained by the increased levels of angiogenic cytokines such as Interleukin-6 (IL-6), TGF-α and TNF-α detected in psoriatic lesions and/or sera. Furthermore, TGF-α stimulates keratinocytes to secrete vascular permeability factor, a selective endothelial cell mitogen that enhances microvascular permeability, two receptors (kdr and flt-1) of which are overexpressed by dermal microvascular endothelial cells in psoriasis.[32]

HEVs are specialised post-capillary venules in which the flat squame-like endothelial cell lining is replaced by that of tall columnar or cuboidal endothelial cells. HEVs are usually restricted to lymphoid tissue but are also found at sites of chronic inflammation or persistent antigenic stimulation such as the dermis in psoriasis[33] and the synovium in rheumatoid arthritis. HEVs play an important role in the recruitment of lymphocytes from the circulation into tissue via the expression of adhesion molecules on both cell types. Indeed, normal or psoriatic blood lymphocytes were shown, in an *in vitro* lymphocyte adherence assay, to bind specifically to dermal microvascular endothelial cells in psoriatic plaques but not to those of uninvolved psoriatic or normal skin. In addition, a preferential binding of CD4+ T cells compared to CD8+ T or B cells was also noted.[34] Expression of adhesion molecules and T cell recruitment to the skin will be discussed in more detail in Chap. 3.

2.7 Neutrophils

Psoriatic lesions are characterised by an infiltration of neutrophils that migrate from the vascular to the dermal compartment and through the layers of the epidermis up to the stratum corneum forming (Munro's) microabscesses. The movement of neutrophils into tissue requires firstly their attachment to endothelial cell walls. An *in vitro* adherence assay designed to measure this function showed that neutrophils from psoriatic patients had increased adherence,[35] and the amount of adherence correlated with disease severity. Several chemotactic factors have been identified in psoriatic lesions which could be responsible for the influx of neutrophils into the epidermis, such as complement fragments, 12-hydroxy-eicosatetraenoic acids and leukotriene-B$_4$. However, the major chemoattractants for neutrophils appear to be members of the C-X-C family, IL-8 and gro-α (see Sec. 6.1.4) and a low molecular mass calcium-binding protein belonging to the S100 family, psoriasin, all of which are highly expressed in the epidermis.[36–38] Furthermore, gro-α has also been detected in the papillary dermis produced by vessel associated cells suggesting that it may also act as an important chemoattractant for neutrophil diapedesis *in vivo*.[37]

Since the expression of these chemokines results from activation of keratinocytes, the infiltration of neutrophils is unlikely to be a primary event in the psoriatic immunopathogenic pathway. Consequently, neutrophils are no longer considered to play a significant role in the psoriatic process.

2.8 Mast Cells

Mast cells containing active tryptase are increased in psoriatic skin lesions and are frequently seen at the basement membrane zone.[39] Furthermore, contacts between mast cells and sensory nerves containing the neuropeptides, Substance P (SP) and calcitonin gene-related peptide (CGRP), are also increased in psoriatic lesions.[40] SP is capable of inducing mast cell degranulation, releasing tryptase which could cleave and activate enzymes known to promote degradation of basement membrane components. This would allow cells and/or mediators easier access to the epidermis to act on keratinocytes, and thus could contribute to keratinocyte hyperproliferation.

Mast cells also interact with dermal dendritic cells which show increased factor XIIIa expression in response to mast cell degranulation, probably resulting from the release of TNF-α.[41] In addition, degranulation of mast cells may also induce the expression of intercellular adhesion molecule-1 (ICAM-1) on psoriatic keratinocytes, probably via the release of TNF-α and histamine.[42]

2.9 Keratinocytes

Epidermal keratinocytes, the other major component of the SIS in psoriasis, are discussed in detail in Chap. 6.

References

1. Streilin J.W. *J.Invest.Dermatol.* **71** (1978), 167–171.
2. Bos J.D. and Kapsenberg M.L. *Immunol.Today* **7** (1986), 235–240.
3. Baker B.S., Swain A.F., Fry L., Valdimarsson H. *Br.J.Dermatol.* **110** (1984), 555–564.
4. Bos J.D. *et al. J.Invest.Dermatol.* **88** (1987), 569–573.
5. Foster C.A. *et al. J.Exp.Med.* **171** (1990), 997–1013.
6. Van der Kerkhof P.C.M., Gerritsen M.J.P., de Jong E.M.G.J. *Clin.Exp.Dermatol.* **21** (1996), 325–329.
7. Bos J.D. *et al. Arch.Dermatol.Res.* **275** (1983), 181–189.
8. Baker B.S. *et al. Clin.Exp.Immunol.* **61** (1985), 526–534.
9. Bos J.D. *et al. Arch.Dermatol.Res.* **281** (1989), 24–30.
10. Bjerke J. *Acta Dermatol.Venereol. (Stockh)* **62** (1982), 477–483.
11. Baker B.S., Swain A.F., Valdimarsson H., Fry L. *Br.J.Dermatol.* **110** (1984), 37–44.
12. Steinman R.M. and Cohn Z.A. *J.Exp.Med.* **137** (1973), 1142–1153.
13. Austyn J.M. *J.Exp.Med.* **183** (1996), 1287–1292.
14. Calabi F. and Milstein C.A. *Nature* **323** (1986), 540–543.
15. Fithian E. *et al. Proc.Natl.Acad.Sci. (USA)* **78** (1981), 2541–2544.
16. Murphy G.F., Branstein B.R., Knowles R.W., Bhan A.K. *Lab.Invest.* **52** (1985), 264–269.
17. Birbeck M.B.C., Breathnach A.S., Everall J.D. *J.Invest.Dermatol.* **37** (1961), 51–54.
18. Poulter L.W., Campbell D.A., Munro C., Janossy G. *Scand.J.Immunol.* **24** (1986), 351–357.
19. Cerio R. *et al. Br.J.Dermatol.* **121** (1989), 421–431.
20. Nestle F.O., Turka L.A., Nickoloff B.J. *J.Clin.Invest.* **94** (1994), 202–209.
21. Mitra R.S. *et al. J.Immunol.* **154** (1995), 2668–2677.
22. Lisi P. *Acta Dermatol.Venereol. (Stockh)* **53** (1973), 425–428.
23. Baker B.S. *et al. Acta Dermatol.Venereol. (Stockh)* **68** (1988), 209–217.
24. Baadsgaard O. *et al. J.Invest.Dermatol.* **92** (1989), 190–195.
25. Cooper K.D., Neises G.R., Katz S.I. *J.Invest.Dermatol.* **86** (1986), 363–370.
26. Bos J.D., van Garderen I.D., Krieg S.R., Poulter L.W. *J.Invest.Dermatol.* **87** (1986), 358–361.
27. Braun-Falco O. and Christophers E. *Arch.Dermatol.Forsch.* **251** (1974), 95–110.

28. Klagsbrun M. *J.Cell Biochem.* **47** (1991), 199–200.
29. de la Brassinne M. and Lachapelle J.M. *Acta Derm.Venereol. (Stockh)* **55** (1975), 171–174.
30. Barton S.P., Abdullah M.S., Marks R. *Br.J.Dermatol.* **126** (1992), 569–574.
31. van de Kerkhof P.C.M., Fleuren E., Van Rennes H., Mier P.D. *Br.J.Dermatol.* **110** (1984), 411–415.
32. Heng M.C.Y., Allen S.G., Chase D.G. *Br.J.Dermatol.* **118** (1988), 315–326.
33. Detmar M. *et al. J.Exp.Med.* **180** (1994), 1141–1146.
34. Sackstein R., Falanga V., Streilein J.W., Chin Y.-H. *J.Invest.Dermatol.* **91** (1988), 423–428.
35. Sedgwick J.B., Bergstresser P.R., Hurd E.R. *J.Invest.Dermatol.* **74** (1980), 81–84.
36. Gillitzer R. *et al. J.Invest.Dermatol.* **97** (1991), 73–79.
37. Gillitzer R. *et al. J.Invest.Dermatol.* **107** (1996), 778–782.
38. Jinquan T. *et al. J.Invest.Dermatol.* **107** (1996), 5–10.
39. Harvima I.T. *et al. Arch.Dermatol.Res.* **282** (1990), 428–433.
40. Naukkarinen A. *et al. J.Pathol.* **180** (1996), 200–205.
41. Sueki H., Whitaker D., Buchsbaum M., Murphy G.F. *Lab.Invest.* **69** (1993), 160–172.
42. Ackermann L. and Harvima I.T. *Arch.Dermatol.Res.* **290** (1998), 353–359.

CHAPTER 3

Immune Cell Function in Psoriasis

3.1 T Lymphocytes: Peripheral Blood

Numbers and ratios of $CD4^+$ and $CD8^+$ T cell subsets in the peripheral blood of patients with psoriasis are generally within normal limits, with the exception of patients with very extensive skin lesions whose systemic $CD4^+$ T cell subpopulation is significantly reduced (Table 3.1).[1,2] This is probably a consequence of the marked infiltration of $CD4^+$ T cells into lesional skin.[2]

Studies of mitogen-induced proliferation of peripheral blood lymphocytes (PBL) in psoriasis have produced conflicting results. Thus, a reduction in PBL response to phytohaemagglutinin (PHA), unrelated to disease activity, was reported by Levantine and Brostoff,[3] whilst Guilhou *et al.* showed a normal response to PHA but significantly reduced proliferation to Concanavalin A (Con A) and pokeweed mitogen.[4] In contrast, another study demonstrated a significantly depressed response to Con A, but normal proliferation to PHA and pokeweed mitogen.[5]

Similar mixed results have come from studies of polyclonal suppressor cell activity in psoriasis. Sauder *et al.*[6] showed that PBL from patients with active psoriasis have a decreased ability to suppress a one-way mixed lymphocyte culture after pre-incubation with Con A for 48 hours. However, Con–A–induced suppressor cell activity, as well as spontaneous suppressor cell function of *in vitro* short-lived adherent cells, were found to be in the normal range

Table 3.1   Blood lymphocyte subpopulations in psoriatic patients. (Source: Baker B.S. *et al. Br.J.Dermatol.* **110 (1984), 37–44, with permission from Blackwell Science Ltd, Oxford, UK.)**

Lymphocyte Population	Controls $n = 28$	Guttate Psoriasis (G) $n = 27$	Chronic Plaque Psoriasis (CP) $n = 24$	Extext of Psoriasis	
				< 10% $n = 37$	> 10% $n = 14$
Total lymphocyte count	2257 ± 99	2055 ± 151	2146 ± 171	2167 ± 122	1915 ± 154
Null	337 ± 49	275 ± 43	‡515 ± 54	360 ± 44	482 ± 77
B	356 ± 31	388 ± 46	340 ± 51	391 ± 43	305 ± 53
T_T	1552 ± 91	1352 ± 106	1307 ± 109	1417 ± 75	†1136 ± 163
% CD4+	65 ± 1.8	65 ± 2.1	65 ± 2.7	65 ± 2.0	61 ± 3.2
CD4+	1021 ± 72	866 ± 76	866 ± 88	927 ± 65	‡706 ± 113
% CD8+	36 ± 0.5	39 ± 2.1	34 ± 2.3	36 ± 1.7	39 ± 3.5
CD8+	557 ± 44	541 ± 55	*432 ± 43	489 ± 39	469 ± 83

Results are expressed as absolute lymphocyte per mm³ ± standard error of the mean (S.E.) CD4+ and CD8+ cells are also expressed as a mean percentage of T_T cells ± s.e.; *n*, number of individuals studied. Significance levels compared with control values: *P = 0.05, †P = 0.02, ‡P < 0.02.

for seven out of eight patients in a second study.[7] A significantly lower suppressor activity in psoriasis patients versus controls was demonstrated using a different approach based on the observation that a significantly higher DNA synthesis is detectable in cultures preincubated for 24 hours at 37°C before stimulation with a suboptimal concentration of Con A than in cultures without preincubation.[8] This increased responsiveness in preincubated cultures is thought to result from a loss of short-lived suppressor cells.

In vivo, patients with psoriasis appear to demonstrate decreased responses to certain antigens which induce delayed hypersensitivity reactions. Thus, although the frequency of positive reactions to 2,4-dinitrochlorobenzene (DNCB) did not differ in psoriatics, the intensity of acquired DNCB sensitization was significantly diminished in the psoriatics compared to controls and appeared to be related to the activity, but not extent of the lesions.[9,10] In addition, psoriatic individuals show a decrease in the amount (not incidence) of both erythema and induration in response to streptokinase/streptodornase (SKSD).[11] Furthermore, a marked delay in resolution of the delayed type hypersensitivity reaction to purified protein derivative (PPD) and, to a lesser extent, SKSD has also been reported.[12]

These findings imply a subtle defect in T lymphocyte function in patients with psoriasis. However, it is unlikely that this represents a primary abnormality but is probably secondary to the disease process.

3.2   T Lymphocytes: Skin

3.2.1   T Cell Homing

In psoriasis as in other inflammatory skin diseases, T lymphocytes are actively recruited into the skin. To gain access to the dermis, T lymphocytes of the memory CD45RO⁺ phenotype expressing lymphocyte function-associated antigen (LFA)-1 (CD11a/CD18) and very late antigen (VLA)-4 (CD49d) integrin receptors must first bind to endothelial cells lining dermal capillary walls via the adhesion molecules intercellular adhesion molecule (ICAM)-1 (CD54) and vascular adhesion molecule (VCAM)-1 (CD106), respectively (Fig. 3.1).

In addition, tissue specificity of T cell egress into the skin is achieved by the expression by T lymphocytes of a skin homing receptor, cutaneous lymphocyte-associated antigen (CLA) which binds to E-selectin (CD62E) on endothelial cells (Fig. 3.1).[13,14]

CLA is expressed on a minor subset of CD45RO⁺ memory T cells in peripheral blood, but by the majority of such cells in cutaneous sites of chronic inflammation such as psoriasis in which E-selectin expression by endothelial cells is upregulated.[13,15] CLA expression is selectively induced on T cells during virgin to memory transition in skin-draining peripheral lymph nodes and is regulated by microenviromental factors such as the cytokine TGFβ₁.[16] In addition, bacterial superantigens (streptococcal and staphylococcal toxins) and group A streptococcal antigens can induce the expansion of skin-homing CLA⁺ T cells via stimulation of IL-12 production.[17,18] In

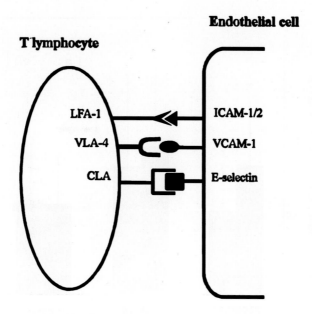

Fig. 3.1. Molecules that mediate adhesion of T lymphocytes to endothelium in skin.

psoriatic patients, but not in normal or disease controls, the streptococcal antigen-induced increase in mean percentage CLA+ expression is significantly greater than that induced by *Candida albicans*, and is accompanied by a decrease in T cells positive for the peripheral lymph node homing receptor, L-selectin (Figs. 3.2 and 3.3).[18] These findings suggest that, in psoriasis, there is a differential modulation of specific tissue homing receptors on T cells by antigens of group A streptococci (GAS), an organism associated with initiation and exacerbation of skin lesions (see Chap. 5).

Recently it has been demonstrated that CLA is an inducible carbohydrate modification of P-selectin glycoprotein ligand (PSGL)-1, a known surface glycoprotein expressed constitutively on all human peripheral blood T cells.[19] Cultured peripheral blood T cells can therefore be differentiated into CLA+ cells which bind both E-selectin and P-selectin, or CLA− cells which bind P-selectin alone, suggesting independent regulation of selectin-binding phenotypes.

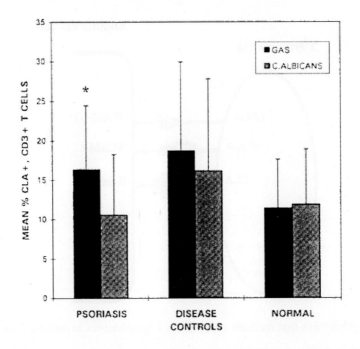

Fig. 3.2. GAS induced a significantly higher increase in CLA$^+$ T cells than *C. albicans* in psoriasis patients. CLA$^+$ T cell expression was analysed after seven days culture of PBMC with GAS (1 µg/ml) or *C. albicans* (100 µg/ml) in 13 psoriasis patients, 10 disease controls and 12 normal individuals. GAS induced significantly higher levels of CLA$^+$ T cells than *C. albicans* in the psoriasis patients only (* p < 0.002). (Source: Baker B.S. *et al.* Induction of cutaneous lymphocyte-associated antigen expression by group A streptococcal antigens in psoriasis, *Arch.Dermatol.Res.* **289** (1997), 671–676, Fig. 2, with permission from Springer-Verlag GmbH & Co, Heidelberg, Germany.)

Furthermore, TH$_1$, but not TH$_2$ cells, (T cell subsets characterised by distinct profiles of cytokine production) are able to bind to both P-selectin and E-selectin and enter into inflamed sites, such as the delayed hypersensitivity reaction to DNFB.[20] This is compatible with the cytokine profile of psoriatic skin T cells which will be discussed in the following section.

Interestingly, it has been shown by two groups that binding of PBL to cultured human umbilical vein endothelium is augmented in

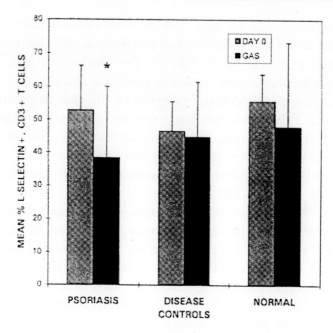

Fig. 3.3. L–selectin T cell expression is reduced by GAS in patients with psoriasis. L–selectin T cell expression was compared in PBMC from 13 psoriasis patients, 10 disease controls and 12 normal controls before and after seven days culture with 1 µg/ml GAS. A significant reduction was observed in the psoriasis patients only (* $p < 0.05$). (Source: Baker B.S. *et al.* Induction of cutaneous lymphocyte-associated antigen expression by group A streptococcal antigens in psoriasis, *Arch.Dermatol. Res.* **289** (1997), 671–676, Fig. 4, with permission from Springer-Verlag GmbH & Co, Heidelberg, Germany.)

patients with psoriasis whilst lymphocytes of patients with atopic dermatitis show decreased binding and those of rheumatoid arthritis patients are no different from that of normal controls.[21,22] This did not appear to be explained by increased T cell expression of LFA-1 or to the presence of serum factors in these patients.[21,22] Similarly, mean CLA expression of freshly isolated psoriatic PBL does not differ from that of patients with other inflammatory skin diseases or normal controls.[18] Thus, the mechanism for augmented lymphocyte binding in patients with psoriasis remains unclear.

It is of relevance in this respect that dermal microvascular endothelial cells from psoriatic, but not normal, skin are resistant to the inhibitory effects by TGF-β_1 on the binding of PBL.[23] These functional alterations may represent part of a mechanism by which T lymphocytes are specifically targeted to the skin in psoriasis.

Once the T lymphocytes have crossed the endothelial barrier and entered the dermis, they interact via integrins with both extracellular matrix components and other cell types such as dermal dendritic cells. In addition, in inflammatory skin disorders, small numbers of mainly CD8[+] T cells pass from the dermis into the epidermis. In psoriasis, this migration is more extensive than in other dermatoses and is, at least partly, a chemotactic response to the high levels of IL-8 produced by keratinocytes in lesional epidermis.[24] Intraepidermal LFA-1[+] T cells then bind and interact with keratinocytes expressing ICAM-1, which is absent from normal epidermis but focally induced by interferon-gamma (IFN-γ) and TNF-α on that of psoriatic lesions.[25]

3.2.2 T Cell Proliferation

T lymphocytes, along with Factor X111a[+] perivascular dendritic cells and endothelial cells, have been shown by immunostaining and autoradiography of ^{3}H-deoxyuridine-injected lesional skin to be proliferating in psoriatic dermis.[26] However, the nature of the stimulating antigen(s) responsible for the activation and subsequent proliferation of the T cell subset capable of inducing the psoriatic lesion remains to be elucidated.

T cell lines (TCL) expanded from biopsies of lesional psoriatic skin in the presence of irradiated, autologous blood lymphocytes and Interleukin-2 (IL-2) have been reported to show autoreactivity, that is, proliferated in culture with autologous PBL.[27] Furthermore, this autoreactivity appeared to be directed against non-HLA antigens, presumably minor HLA antigens, because the cell lines giving rise to a positive response did not share a particular HLA specificity that was absent on those that did not.[27] However, it has been observed that T cell clones isolated from psoriatic skin are commonly highly reactive to autologous cells when first isolated but lose this autoreactivity after freezing and subsequent thawing[28] casting doubt on the relevance of the above findings.

In a more recent study in which T cells were expanded from psoriatic skin lesions in an antigen-independent fashion to avoid skewing of T cell subpopulations towards responsiveness to any specific antigen, a lack of reactivity to a range of epidermal antigen preparations was demonstrated.[29] However, since T cells specific for the putative psoriasis antigen(s) are likely to be present as a small proportion of an infiltrate of predominately non-specifically recruited T cells, it seems probable that the authors would have been more likely to detect such cells if they had been expanded out in the presence of specific antigen. This latter approach was used in two earlier studies which successfully demonstrated T cell reactivity to two different organisms that are associated clinically with psoriasis.[30,31]

TCL from skin lesions of five patients with guttate psoriasis responded strongly to heat-killed and sonicated group A streptococci of three different M serotypes, whilst control TCL generated from patients with other inflammatory skin diseases showed lower and less frequent responses (Tables 3.2 and 3.3).[30]

Clones were established from one of these psoriatic TCL (NY); eight of the nine T cell clones were found to respond to streptococcal antigens (Fig. 3.4). Of these, four were stable and responded in an HLA-restricted fashion to one or more of the streptococcal preparations.[30] It has been shown subsequently that streptococcal antigen-reactive TCL can also be isolated from skin lesions of CP psoriasis[31] implicating a role for this organism in both initiation and maintenance of the psoriatic process (see Chap. 5 for a detailed discussion).

In addition, T cells showing a differential reactivity to *Pityrosporum orbiculare* versus *Pityrosporum ovale* have been cultured from scalp

Table 3.2   Proliferative responses of skin T cell lines from patients with guttate psoriasis, eczema, lichen planus and pityriasis rosea to Strep-A1, A2 and A3. (Source: Baker B.S. *et al. Br.J.Dermatol.* **128 (1993), 493–499, with permission from Blackwell Science Ltd, Oxford, UK.)**

	A1	A2	A3
Guttate psoriasis			
NY	**45,805** (3,845)	NR	**4,267** (803)
MC	**33,305** (268)	**21,487** (2,588)	**32,182** (666)
GR	NR	**4,759** (506)	**11,779** (187)
EH	NR	**2,180** (75)	**16,519** (400)
MA	**19,667** (8,753)	**38,097** (1,384)	**45,082** (1,993)
Eczema			
1	NR	NR	NR
2	NR	**1,427** (266)	NR
3	**2,951** (726)	**25,832** (2,753)	**9,161** (5,692)
4	NR	NR	NR
5	NR	1,155	NR
Lichen planus			
1	NR	NR	NR
2	NR	NR	NR
3	NR	**10,563** (2,180)	**7,899** (1,076)
4	**8,758** (411)	**18,748** (1,744)	**3,304** (2,039)
5	NR	NR	NR
Pityriasis rosea			
1	**1,630** (367)	NR	NR
2	**12,093** (2,261)	NR	NR

Data are expressed as mean c.p.m. of TCL in the presence of antigen minus TCL in the absence of antigen. Background counts of TCLs in the absence of antigen ranged from 35–2,953 c.p.m. Standard deviations are shown in parentheses, responses > 1,000 c.p.m. are in bold. NR, no responses (< 1,000 c.p.m.).

Table 3.3   Proliferative responses of skin T cell lines from lesions of nickel contact dermatitis and PPD-induced DTH responses to Strep-A1, A2 and A3. (Source: Baker B.S. *et al. Br.J.Dermatol.* 128 (1993), 493–499, with permission from Blackwell Science Ltd, Oxford, UK.)

	A1	A2	A3	Ni	PPD
Nickel CD					
1	NR	NR	NR	**30,541** (4,129)	ND
2	**2,846** (2,393)	NR	NR	**25,759** (3,001)	ND
3	**1,153** (280)	NR	NR	**7,371** (1,289)	ND
PPD DTH					
1	**2,482** (986)	NR	NR	ND	**86,909** (4,026)
2	**5,265** (974)	NR	NR	ND	**108,333** (4,856)
3	NR	NR	NR	ND	**60,092** (5,083)

Data are expressed as mean c.p.m. of the TCL in the presence of antigen minus TCL in the absence of antigen. (Background counts of TCLs in the absence of antigen ranged from 45 to 3,147). Standard deviations are shown in parentheses, responses > 1,000 c.p.m. are in bold. Concentrations/dillutions of antigens used were Strep-A1, 1 μg/ml; Strep-A2, 1 : 10,000; Strep-A3, 1 : 10,000; nickel sulphate, 5×10^{-5} M; PPD, 100 U/ml. NR, no response (defined as < 1,000 c.p.m.); ND, not done.

(and non-scalp) lesions of CP psoriasis (Fig. 3.5).[32] T cells with similar reactivity have been isolated from scalp lesions of alopecia areata indicating that T cell recognition of *Pityrosporum* is not psoriasis-specific. Thus, sensitized T cells appear to home to sites such as the scalp where the organism forms part of the normal skin flora. However, both the frequency and degree of response to *Pityrosporum* by scalp T cells were substantially lower in the alopecia areata compared to psoriatic patients suggesting that these cells could play a role in the pathogenesis of psoriasis. Differences in antigenic determinants recognised, pattern of cytokines produced, regulatory T cell function and/or the response of KC to T cell-derived factors could conceivably lead to the initiation of the psoriatic process by *Pityrosporum*-reactive T cells in genetically predisposed individuals.

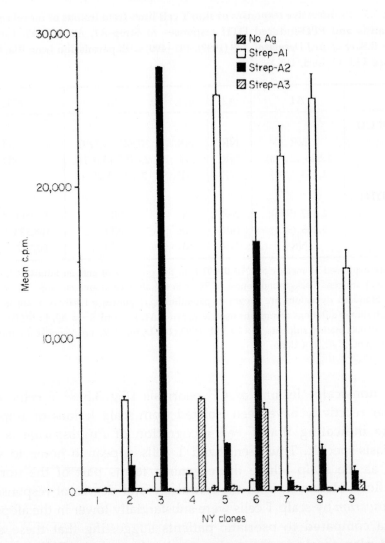

Fig. 3.4. Proliferation of NY skin T cell clones to Strep-A1, A2 and A3. Strep-A1 is a mixture of four isolates: one M4, two M12, and one untyped). Strep-A2 and A3 are single isolates expressing M22 and M1 antigens respectively. Data are expressed as mean cpm (three replicates); bars show standard deviation. (Source: Baker B.S. *et al. Br.J.Dermatol.* **128** (1993), 493–499, with permission from Blackwell Science Ltd, Oxford, UK.)

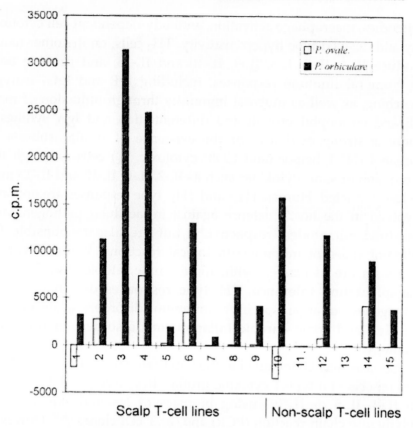

Fig. 3.5. Increased proliferative response by lesional scalp (1–9) and non-scalp (10–15) TCL to *P.orbiculare* compared to *P.ovale* cytoplasmic extracts in patients with psoriasis. Background cpm in the absence of antigen have been subtracted (61–4, 416). (Source: Baker B.S. *et al. Br.J.Dermatol.* **136** (1997), 319–325, with permission from Blackwell Science Ltd, Oxford, UK.)

3.2.3 *Cytokine Production*

CD4+ T cells can be subdivided into functional subsets (TH$_1$ and TH$_2$) based upon their cytokine profiles. This was first described for murine T cell clones.[33] TH$_1$ cells produce IFN-γ, IL-2 and TNF-β, and promote the production of opsonising and complement-fixing antibodies, macrophage activation, antibody-dependent cell cytotoxicity and delayed-type hypersensitivity. TH_2 cells, on the other hand, produce IL-4, IL-5, Il-6, IL-9, IL-10 and IL-13, and provide help for humoral immune responses, including IgE and IgG_1 isotype switching, as well as mucosal immunity through induction of mast cell and eosinophil growth and differentiation and IgA synthesis. There is strong evidence for the existence of similar subsets of human CD4$^+$ T helper (and CD8$^+$ cytotoxic, T_c) cells although the expression of some cytokines such as IL-2, IL-6, IL-10 and IL-13 may be less restricted. Human TH_1- and TH_2- type responses are not only involved in the host's defence against intracellular pathogens and intestinal nematodes, respectively, but are also responsible for different types of immunopathological reactions. Whilst TH_2-type responses are associated with, for example, atopic disorders and transplantation tolerance, TH_1-type responses dominate in the pathogenesis of organ-specific autoimmune disorders, acute allograft rejection and some chronic inflammatory disorders of unknown aetiology.[34]

Psoriasis may be included in the latter category as there have been two reports of a type 1 cytokine profile (IL-2, IFN-γ and TNF-α, but no IL-4, IL-5 or IL-10) using biopsies of lesional skin and the polymerase chain reaction (PCR) and/or T cell clones.[35,36] However, a further study of the cytokine mRNA profile expressed in lesional psoriatic skin and in T cell clones established from skin lesions revealed a cytokine pattern distinct from that of TH_1- or TH_2- type cells.[37] Thus, in addition to TH_1-type cytokines, IFN-γ and IL-2, TH_2-type cytokine IL-5, but not IL-4, was also present.[37] Furthermore, those psoriatic T cell clones producing this combination of cytokines, but not those with TH_0 or TH_1 cytokine profiles, yielded supernatants mitogenic for keratinocytes *in vitro*.[37]

The factors in T cell-conditioned media which stimulate keratinocyte proliferation have not yet been identified,[38,39] but depend upon the presence of IFN-γ since neutralisation of the latter cytokine with specific antibody abolished mitogenic activity.[38]

3.3 Antigen-Presenting Cells

3.3.1 *Epidermal Dendritic Cells*

The stimulatory capacity of epidermal dendritic cells, compared to peripheral blood APC, appears to be altered in psoriasis. Thus lesional psoriatic epidermal cells show an increased capacity to induce allogeneic T cell activation and proliferation compared to those from uninvolved psoriatic skin.[40] Furthermore, both lesional and uninvolved psoriatic epidermal cells are more active in stimulating autologous T cell proliferation than cells from the epidermis of normal individuals and/or lichen planus and contact allergy patients.[41,42] However, in an earlier study autologous uninvolved psoriatic epidermal cells showed poor stimulation of T cells in common with those isolated from normal skin.[43]

In both autologous and allogeneic T cell activation by psoriatic epidermal cells, the principal stimulator cells involved were shown to be those of the HLA-DR$^+$/CD1a$^-$ subset.[40,42] Because the phenotype and some functional characteristics of cultured LC and HLA-DR$^+$/CD1a$^-$ APC are similar, it has been proposed that the epidermal dendritic cells in a psoriatic lesion may resemble those of lymph nodes, that is, mature cells that can initiate primary T cell immune reactions.[44]

3.3.2 *Dermal Dendritic Cells (DDC)*

In common with epidermal dendritic cells, DDC from lesional psoriatic skin have an increased ability to stimulate autologous T cell proliferation compared to psoriatic blood-derived dendritic cells or those from normal skin.[45] Antibody blocking studies revealed the involvement of HLA-DR, B7 and LFA-1 expressed on lesional DDC in the induction of the T cell response, which was characterised by the production of high levels of IL-2 and IFN-γ (TH$_1$-type), but no IL-4 or IL-10 (TH$_2$-type).[46] DDC derived from normal skin produced a similar pattern of cytokines but in lower quantities.

Psoriatic DDC have also been shown to act as potent APCs for allogeneic T cell responses.[46] Interactions between DDC and T cells have been blocked almost completely by CTLA-4Ig, a potent inhibitor of CD28-mediated pathways that can block both B7-1 (CD80) and B7-2 (CD86) binding to CD28.[45,46]

References

1. DePietro W.P., Berger C.L., Harber L.C., Edelson R.L. *J.Am.Acad.Dermatol.* **5** (1981), 304–307.
2. Baker B.S., Swain A.F., Valdimarsson H., Fry L. *Br.J.Dermatol.* **110** (1984), 37–44.
3. Levantine A. and Brostoff J. *Br.J.Dermatol.* **93** (1975), 659–666.
4. Guilhou J.J. *et al. Br.J.Dermatol.* **95** (1976), 295–301.
5. Clot J., Dardenne M., Bouchier J. *Clin.Immunol.Immunopathol.* **9** (1978), 389–397.
6. Sauder D.N., Bailin P.L., Sundeen J., Krakauer R.S. *Arch.Dermatol.* **116** (1980), 51–55.
7. Clot J., Guilhou J.J., Andary M. *J.Invest.Dermatol.* **78** (1982), 313–315.
8. Hunyadi J., Dobozy A., Kenderessy A.Sz., Simon N. *J.Invest.Dermatol.* **75** (1980), 217–218.
9. Glinski W. *et al. J.Invest.Dermatol.* **70** (1978), 105–110.
10. Obalek S., Haftek M., Glinski W. *Dermatologica* **155** (1977), 13–23.
11. Krueger G.G., Hill H.R., Jederberg W.W. *J.Invest.Dermatol.* **71** (1978), 189–194.
12. McFadden J.P. *et al. Acta Dermatol.Venereol. (Stockh)* **70** (1989), 262–264.
13. Picker L.J., Michie S.A., Rott L.S., Butcher E.C. *Am.J.Pathol.* **136** (1990), 1053–1068.
14. Picker L.J. *et al. Nature* **349** (1991), 796–811.
15. Picker L.J. *et al. Eur.J.Immunol.* **24** (1994), 1269–1277.
16. Picker L.J. *et al. J.Immunol.* **150** (1993), 1122–1136.
17. Leung D.Y.M. *et al. J.Exp.Med.* **181** (1995), 747–753.
18. Baker B.S. *et al. Arch.Dermatol.Res.* **289** (1997), 671–676.
19. Fuhlbrigge R.C., Kieffer J.D., Armerding D., Kupper T.S. *Nature* **389** (1997), 978–981.
20. Austrop F. *et al. Nature* **385** (1997), 81–83.

21. LeRoy F. *et al.* *J.Invest.Dermatol.* **97** (1991), 511–516.
22. Lee M.L. *et al.* *Clin.Exp.Immunol.* **91** (1993), 346–350.
23. Cai J.P., Falanga V., Taylor J.R., Chin Y.H. *J.Invest.Dermatol.* **98** (1992), 405–409.
24. Sticherling M., Bornscheuer E., Schroder J.M., Christophers E. *J.Invest. Dermatol.* **96** (1991), 26–30.
25. Griffiths C.E.M., Voorhees J.J., Nickoloff B.J. *J.Am.Acad.Dermatol.* **20** (1989), 617–629
26. Morganroth G.S. *et al.* *J.Invest.Dermatol.* **96** (1991), 333–340.
27. Nikaein A. *et al.* *J.Invest.Dermatol.* **96** (1991), 3–9.
28. Baker B.S. and Fry L. *J.Invest.Dermatol.* **97** (1991), 606.
29. Horrocks C., Holder J.E., Berth-Jones J., Camp R.D.R. *Br.J.Dermatol.* **137** (1997), 331–338.
30. Baker B.S. *et al.* *Br.J.Dermatol.* **128** (1993), 493–499.
31. Baker B.S. *et al.* *Arch.Dermatol.Res.* (1999), (in press).
32. Baker B.S. *et al.* *Br.J.Dermatol.* **136** (1997), 319–325.
33. Mosmann T.R. *et al.* *J.Immunol.* **136** (1986), 2348–2357.
34. Romagnani S. *Clin.Immunol.Immunopathol.* **80** (1996), 225–235.
35. Uyemura K. *et al.* *J.Invest.Dermatol.* **101** (1993), 701–705.
36. Schlaak J.F. *et al.* *J.Invest.Dermatol.* **102** (1994), 145–149.
37. Vollmer S. *et al.* *Eur.J.Immunol.* **24** (1994), 2377–2382.
38. Prinz J.C. *et al.* *Eur.J.Immunol.* **24** (1994), 593–598.
39. Strange P. *et al.* *J.Invest.Dermatol.* **101** (1993), 695–700,
40. Baadsgaard O. *et al.* *J.Invest.Dermatol.* **92** (1989), 190–195.
41. Steinmuller D., Zinsmeister A.R., Rogers R.S. *J.Autoimm.* **1** (1988), 279–298.
42. Prens E.P., Benne K., van Joost T., Benner R. *J.Invest.Dermatol.* **96** (1991), 880–887.
43. Schopf R.E. *et al.* *Arch.Dermatol.Res.* **279** (1986), 89–94.
44. Streilein J.W. *J.Invest.Dermatol.* **95** (1990), 20S–21S.
45. Nestle F.O., Turka L.A., Nickoloff B.J. *J.Clin.Invest.* **94** (1994), 202–209.
46. Nestle F.O. *et al.* *Cell.Immunol.* **156** (1994), 220–229.

CHAPTER 4

Psoriasis is a T Cell-Mediated Disease

As described in Chap. 2, early studies showed an association between clinical activity and the phenotype of T cell subpopulations present in guttate psoriatic lesions. Thus, the eruption of acute skin lesions coincided with the epidermal influx and activation of CD4$^+$ T cells whereas disease resolution was associated with recruitment and activation of CD8$^+$ T cells.

This was followed up by various investigations designed to determine the extent of involvement of T lymphocytes in the immunopathogenesis of psoriasis. This included the use of various immunosuppressive treatments including cyclosporin A (CyA) and FK506, anti-CD4 monoclonal antibodies and lymphocyte-selective toxin (DAB$_{389}$IL-2) to clear psoriasis, the dermal injection of immuno-cytes into Severe Combined Immunodeficient (SCID) mice to induce psoriasis, transfer or resolution of the disease by bone-marrow transplantation, and the promotion of keratinocyte proliferation by supernatants from T cell clones isolated from psoriatic skin lesions.

The results from these studies provide compelling evidence for the notion that psoriasis is a T cell-mediated disease.

4.1 Anti-Psoriatic Treatments

Resolution of CP lesions during treatment with topical steroids, psoralens plus UVA light (PUVA) or dithranol (a synthetic analogue

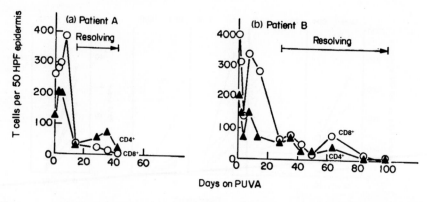

Fig. 4.1. Marked reduction of epidermal T cells precedes resolution in patient A who responded early, and patient B who responded slowly to PUVA treatment. ▲ CD4⁺ T; o CD8⁺ T; HPF = high power fields. (Source: Baker B.S. *et al. Clin.Exp.Immunol.* **61** (1985), 526–534, with permission from Blackwell Science Ltd, Oxford, UK.)

of the natural substance chrysarobin) is accompanied by depletion of both epidermal and dermal CD4⁺ and CD8⁺ T cells.[1,2] The rate of disappearance of both cell types in the epidermis correlates with the rate of resolution in individual patients and, in PUVA-treated patients, the depletion of epidermal T cells precedes the onset of clinical improvement (Fig. 4.1).

On the basis of these, and previous findings, it was postulated that psoriasis is a disease of abnormal keratinocyte proliferation induced by T cells.[3] This hypothesis predicted that the immuno-suppressive drug CyA, whose primary action is the selective inhibition of cytokine production by CD4⁺ T cells, should be effective in clearing psoriasis. Subsequent studies confirmed that this was indeed the case and that, furthermore, the macrolide antibiotic FK506 which shares a number of immunosuppressive properties with CyA also proved to be a potent anti-psoriatic agent.[4,5]

Resolution of psoriasis by treatment with CyA was accompanied by a decrease in CD4⁺ and CD8⁺ T cells. However HLA-DR⁺ CD4⁺ T cells persisted in the epidermis of resolved lesions (Fig. 4.2).[6]

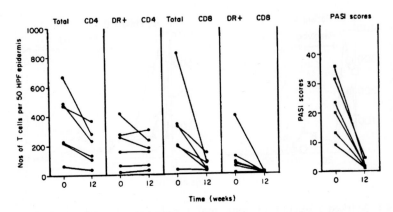

Fig. 4.2. Numbers and HLA-DR expression of T lymphocytes in the lesional epidermis of six psoriasis patients before and after 12 weeks treatment with CyA. HPF = high power fields; PASI = Psoriasis Area and Severity Index. (Source: Baker B.S. *et al.* *Br.J.Dermatol.* **116** (1987), 503–510, with permission from Blackwell Science Ltd, Oxford, UK.)

These activated epidermal CD4[+] T cells disappeared when CyA was injected intradermally into the skin lesion suggesting that a higher local concentration of the drug was required to deplete this subpopulation.[7] FK506 also induced a rapid disappearance of the inflammatory infiltrate which was followed by a slower resolution of the epidermal changes.[5]

It should be pointed out that the effects of some of these immunosuppressive treatments are not confined to T lymphocytes and that their modulation of APC cell numbers and/or function probably also contributes to their efficacy in clearing psoriasis. Thus, PUVA and topical steroids reduce the numbers of LC in psoriatic epidermis, although this occurs subsequent to the marked depletion of T cells.[1,2] Interestingly, dithranol and CyA selectively decrease only the HLA-DR[+], CD1a[-] subpopulation of LC whilst total numbers of dendritic cells are largely unaffected.[2,6] Furthermore, a delayed inhibition of LC-mediated activation of T cells by CyA, which appears to correlate with the time course and level of reduction in non-LC, HLA-DR[+] leukocytes, has also been reported in psoriasis.[8]

The possibility that CyA acts directly on keratinocyte function in psoriasis has also been addressed. Inhibition of keratinocyte proliferation induced by CyA has been reported under culture conditions in which calcium levels are low and serum is absent.[9] The relevance of these observations is, therefore, questionable due to the unphysiological nature of the culture conditions. On the other hand, it is possible that CyA may inhibit keratinocyte proliferation indirectly by blocking keratinocyte production of cytokines stimulatory for their own growth.

Urabe *et al.* have reported inhibition of keratinocyte proliferation by CyA *in vivo* using human skin grafted onto nude, athymic mice.[10] They were unable to demonstrate the presence of human T cells in the grafts and therefore attributed the inhibition to a direct effect of the drug on keratinocytes. However, it has been shown that psoriatic skin grafts on nude, athymic mice are infiltrated with activated mouse T cells which potentially could secrete cytokines capable of stimulating human epidermal cell growth.[11] CyA could therefore conceivably act on these mouse T cells thereby inhibiting proliferation of the epidermal layer of the grafted skin. Thus, the evidence for a direct action by CyA on keratinocyte proliferation is not convincing. FK506 has been shown to have no direct effect.[12] A more detailed description of the mechanism of action of various immunosuppressive treatments used in psoriasis is given in Chap. 7.

4.2 Anti-CD4 Monoclonal Antibodies

A genetically engineered chimaeric human/mouse CD4 monoclonal antibody injected intravenously into a patient with generalised pustular psoriasis proved to have a potent anti-psoriatic effect which was accompanied by a decrease in the CD4$^+$ T cell count and loss of T cells from lesional skin.[13] Similar findings were obtained in a second study of three patients with severe psoriasis given a murine CD4 monoclonal antibody for seven or eight days; rapid clinical improvement was observed during one month after treatment.[14]

However, IgM and/or IgG antibodies were produced against the anti-CD4 monoclonal antibody at days seven to eight or 15 in all three patients.

4.3 Lymphocyte-Selective Toxin (DAB$_{389}$IL-2)

To address the role of T cells in psoriasis, a fusion protein in which the receptor binding domain of diphtheria toxin was replaced by human IL-2 and the membrane-translocating and cytotoxic domains were retained (DAB$_{389}$IL-2) was used.[15] Studies in experimental and clinical IL-2 receptor-expressing lymphomas have demonstrated that this toxin allows the selective elimination of cells expressing IL-2 receptors. In the case of psoriatic skin lesions, this would target the toxins to activated T cells but would leave keratinocytes, which lack IL-2 receptors, unaffected. Out of the ten patients with chronic, extensive plaque psoriasis who were administered the toxin, four showed striking clinical improvement, four had moderate improvement and two had minimal improvement after two cycles of treatment.

This clinical response correlated with changes in epidermal activation and T cell infiltration in skin lesions.[15] Thus numbers of infiltrating T cells were reduced in both epidermis and dermis in all patients but the most marked reductions were observed in the four patients with the most striking clinical improvement. The reversal of several molecular markers of epidermal dysfunction was associated with a marked reduction in intraepidermal CD3$^+$ or CD8$^+$ T cells.

This study clearly supports the concept that T cells are central to the pathogenesis of psoriasis.

4.4 SCID Mouse Models

Investigations of the mechanisms involved in the psoriatic pathogenic process have been hampered by the lack of a suitable animal model. When psoriatic lesional skin was tranplanted onto athymic, nude mice, human lymphocytes disappeared from such grafts within 48 hours and the latter become infiltrated with Thy 1.2[+] mouse lymphocytes.[11] More recently, Nickoloff et al.[16] have reported the development of a new animal model in which normal or psoriatic skin is transplanted onto SCID mice which, unlike athymic, nude mice, do not possess T lymphocytes. They showed that the transplanted human skin grafts had excellent acceptance rates, and retention of clinical, histological and immunological phenotype characteristics. Furthermore, when autologous, blood-derived immunocytes (a mixture of lymphocytes and monocytes) were injected into the dermis of transplanted uninvolved psoriatic skin, conversion to a fully-fledged psoriatic plaque was observed on each of the ten occasions involving skin from six different psoriatic patients.[17] However, none of four normal skin samples injected with autologous immunocytes also converted to psoriatic plaques. With one exception, the immunocytes required preactivation with IL-2 and superantigens for the conversion to take place. However, stimulation of subpopulations of T cells expressing a particular Vβ family does not appear to be required since PHA-activated immunocytes give the same results as those activated by the superantigens Staphylococcal exotoxin-B and -C_2 (SEB, SEC_2) (Nickoloff B.J., personal communication).

This study has, however, left unanswered whether activated immunocytes from a non-psoriatic individual would induce a similar conversion of uninvolved to lesional psoriatic skin. Conversely, the authors report that one out of four normal skin grafts injected with allogeneic cells from a psoriatic patient developed psoriasis. Since the genes for psoriasis are common in the community, it is possible that the skin that converted came from a genetically predisposed individual who has yet to present with the disease. If so, this would provide further support for the additional involvement of a keratinocyte functional defect in the pathogenic process.

Similarly, another group reported that when clinically uninvolved skin from psoriasis patients was grafted onto SCID mice and injected with superantigen exfoliative toxin from *Staphylococcus aureus*, some histological and immunohistological features of psoriasis were induced.[18] Furthermore, when superantigen-stimulated PBMC from psoriasis patients were simultaneously administered intraperitoneally, homing of CLA+ T cells to graft epidermis was observed. This phenomenon was an exclusive feature of psoriatic skin plus PBMC.

A different approach was used by Gilhar *et al.*[19] who transplanted lesional rather than uninvolved psoriatic skin onto SCID mice and observed that it gradually lost many of its psoriatic features. However, injection (intravenous or intradermal) of autologous cultured skin-infiltrating T cells, but not of autologous cultured PBMC, prevented these changes and maintained the psoriatic phenotype including epidermal acanthosis, elevated labelling index, etc. In contrast, injection of autologous skin-infiltrating T cells into normal skin from non-psoriatic donors had no effect on either epidermal thickness or labelling index. Although it was stated that T cells from all sources were cultured with IL-2 and similarly activated, skin T cells would actually be in a more activated state than those from peripheral blood with higher expression of molecules such as CLA and IL-2 receptor. This would be analogous to superantigen-stimulated PBMC employed in the previous two studies.[17,18]

The findings obtained with this animal model clearly support the idea that psoriasis is mediated by blood- or skin-derived immunocytes which, once activated and present in the skin, secondarily induce keratinocyte and endothelial cell proliferation.

4.5 Bone-Marrow Transplantation

The first clinical case report of the transfer of psoriasis by allogeneic bone-marrow transplantation was reported in 1990 in a patient who had no previous history of the disease.[20] The onset of the disease was delayed by six months which may be due to the immunosuppressive drug regime used for prophylaxis and treatment of Graft versus Host disease (GVHD). Thus psoriasis developed despite the patient's treatment with CyA at a dose used to effectively clear skin lesions.

In a second case report, a patient was described in whom the development of psoriasis occurred shortly after receiving syngeneic bone-marrow from his psoriatic twin.[21] Furthermore, psoriasis recurred with arthropathy following a second syngeneic bone-marrow transplantation.[21]

Conversely, clearance of severe psoriasis following allogeneic bone-marrow transplantation from non-psoriatic individuals has also been reported.[22,23] This remission is long-standing in the absence of immunosuppression. Thus, replacement of a psoriatic patient's bone-marrow-derived immune system with that of a genetically different, non-psoriatic donor appears to bring about total remission pointing to a central role for marrow-derived lymphocytes in the pathogenesis of psoriasis. However, it is not known what the relative contribution of intensive immunosuppression might have been on the inhibition of the psoriatic process.

4.6 T Cell Supernatants Promote Keratinocyte Proliferation

As previously mentioned in Chap. 3, supernatants from T cell clones isolated from psoriatic skin lesions have been shown to stimulate growth of normal keratinocytes *in vitro*.[24,25] Mitogenic activity was largely abolished by addition of antiserum to IFN-γ, but as IFN-γ alone is a potent inhibitor of normal keratinocyte growth, the ultimate effect appears to be decided by the presence of additional cytokines.[24] Of relevance in this context is the finding that keratinocytes from lesional psoriatic skin are much less responsive to inhibition by IFN-γ[26] and that, furthermore, intradermal injection of recombinant IFN-γ can result in the induction of a psoriatic lesion.[27] Thus, the T cell-derived cytokine IFN-γ appears to be a key component of the psoriatic process.

Further evidence for the involvement of T cells in the pathogenesis of psoriasis is the finding that basal and suprabasal keratinocytes express CDw60 in lesional but not in normal epidermis, and that soluble factors derived from lesional T cells induce the expression of CDw60 on normal keratinocytes.[28] Both IL-4 and IL-13 can strongly upregulate CDw60; anti-IL-13 (but not anti-IL-4) partially neutralised the upregulation of CDw60 by the T cell supernatants.[28] Thus, the effect of T cell supernatants on expression of CDw60 on keratinocytes is partly due to IL-13, a TH_2-type cytokine.

Antibodies to CDw60 are mitogenic for preactivated T cells implicating this molecule as a costimulator for T cell activation. The role of CDw60 on keratinocytes is, however, unknown. Its upregulation on hyperproliferating cells in basal cell carcinoma suggests that it may be involved in proliferation of not only T cells, but of keratinocytes as well.

4.7 Low CD4+/HIV Infection

The induction and exacerbation of psoriasis in patients with HIV infection has been used as evidence to contradict the notion that psoriasis is mediated by T cells. Examination of psoriatic skin lesions from patients with AIDS showed that CD8+ T cells predominated in the dermis, a reversal of the ratio in non-AIDS psoriasis.[29] However, by analogy to a delayed-type hypersensitivity (DTH) response to a contact allergen in the skin, only a very small number of antigen-specific CD4+ T cells would be required to initiate the psoriatic process. AIDS patients who still possess circulating CD4+ T cells would, therefore, potentially be able to develop psoriasis, but the skin lesions would be expected to clear when peripheral CD4+ T cells are depleted in the terminal stages of the disease.

Interestingly a patient with a profound CD4+ lymphocytopenia and widespread, recalcitrant psoriasis, who was found negative for the HIV virus, was shown to have similar numbers of activated CD4+ T cells in lesional epidermis as a group of patients with normal circulating CD4+ T cell counts, although total numbers of epidermal CD4+ T cells were decreased.[30] In contrast, total and HLA-DR+ epidermal CD8+ T cell numbers were greatly increased (Table 4.1).

Table 4.1   Total and HLA-DR⁺, CD4⁺ and CD8⁺ T cell numbers
in the epidermis and dermis of a CD4⁺ lymphocytopenic
psoriasis patient: comparison with previously reported data.[1]
Counts per 50 high power fields of epidermis; counts per
section of dermis. % HLA-DR⁺ T cell are shown in parentheses.
(Source: Hardman C.M. *et al. Br.J.Dermatol.* 136 (1997),
930–932, with permission from Blackwell Science Ltd, Oxford,
UK.)

	CD4⁺ Lymphocytopenic Patient		Patient with Psoriasis (n = 17)	
	Total	HLA-DR⁺	Total	HLA-DR⁺
Epidermis				
CD4⁺	36	22 (61)	199 ± 21	32 (16)
CD8⁺	633	315 (50)	365 ± 44	33 (9)
CD4⁺/CD8⁺	0.06	0.07	0.66 ± 0.10	0.97
Dermis				
CD4⁺	170	158 (93)	204 ± 24	106 (52)
CD8⁺	133	76 (57)	119 ± 18	38 (32)
CD4⁺/CD8⁺	1.28	2.08	2.05 ± 0.26	2.79

Thus, a substantial decrease in circulating CD4⁺ T cells does not
prevent the induction of psoriasis. On the contrary, the process
appears more activated. This may be explained by an increased
contribution by activated CD8⁺ T cells, which predominate in these
cases, to the psoriatic process perhaps via the release of cytokines
such as IFN-γ. The demonstration that epidermal CD8⁺ T cells in CP
lesions preferentially express Vβ3 and/or Vβ13.1, and furthermore,
show mono- or oligo-clonality which persists over several months,
supports this idea.[31]

References

1. Baker B.S. *et al. Clin.Exp.Immunol.* **61** (1985), 526–534.
2. Baker B.S. *et al. Scand.J.Immunol.* **22** (1985), 471–477.

3. Valdimarsson H., Baker B.S., Jonsdottir I., Fry L. *Immunol.Today* **7** (1986), 256–259.
4. Griffiths C.E.M. *et al. Br.Med.J.* **293** (1986), 731–732.
5. Ackerman C. *et al. J.Invest.Dermatol.* **96** (1991), 536 (Abstract).
6. Baker B.S. *et al. Br.J.Dermatol.* **116** (1987), 503–510.
7. Baker B.S. *et al. Br.J.Dermatol.* **120** (1989), 207–213.
8. Cooper K.D. *et al. J.Invest.Dermatol.* **94** (1990), 649–656.
9. Nickoloff B.J., Fisher G.J., Mitra R.S., Voorhees J.J. *Am.J.Pathol.* **131** (1988), 12–18.
10. Urabe A., Kanitakis J., Viac J., Thivolet J. *J.Invest.Dermatol.* **92** (1989), 755–757.
11. Baker B.S. *et al. Br.J.Dermatol.* **126** (1992), 105–110.
12. Somach S., Hebda P., Warty V., Jeyasothy B. *J.Invest.Dermatol.* **96** (1991), 580 (Abstract).
13. Prinz J. *et al. Lancet* **338** (1991), 320–321.
14. Morel P. *et al. J.Autoimmun.* **5** (1992), 465–477.
15. Gottlieb S.L. *et al. Nat.Med.* **1** (1995), 442–447.
16. Nickoloff B.J., Kunkel S.L., Burdick M., Strieter R.M. *Am.J.Pathol.* **146** (1995), 580–588.
17. Wrone-Smith T. and Nickoloff B.J. *J.Clin.Invest.* **98** (1996), 1878–1887.
18. Boehncke W.H., Dressel D., Zollner T.M., Kaufmann R. *Nature* **379** (1996), 777 (letter).
19. Gilhar A. *et al. J.Invest.Dermatol.* **109** (1997), 283–288.
20. Gardembas-Pain M. *et al. Arch.Dermatol.* **126** (1990), 1523.
21. Snowden J.A. and Heaton D.C. *Br.J.Dermatol.* **137** (1997), 130–132.
22. Eedy D.J., Burrows D., Bridges J.M., Jones F.G.C. *Br.Med.J.* **300** (1990), 908.
23. Jowitt S.N. and Jal Y. *Br.Med.J.* **300** (1990), 1398–1399.
24. Prinz J.C. *et al. Eur.J.Immunol.* **24** (1994), 593–598.
25. Strange P. *et al. J.Invest.Dermatol.* **101** (1993), 695–700.
26. Baker B.S., Powles A.V., Valdimarsson H., Fry L. *Scand.J.Immunol.* **28** (1988), 735–740.
27. Fierlbeck G., Rasner G., Muler G. *Arch.Dermatol.* **126** (1990), 315–325.
28. Skov L. *et al. Am.J.Pathol.* **150** (1997), 675–683.
29. Steigleder G.K., Rasokat H., Wemmer U. *Z.Hautkr.* **61** (1986), 1671–1678.
30. Hardman C.M. *et al. Br.J.Dermatol.* **136** (1997), 930–932.
31. Chang J.C.C. *et al. Proc.Natl.Acad.Sci. (USA)* **91** (1994), 9282–9286.

β Haemolytic Streptococci and Psoriasis

The nature of the antigen(s) that activates T lymphocytes in psoriasis has remained undetermined. However, it has been well documented that infections of the upper respiratory tract, particularly those induced by β haemolytic streptococci, are associated with acute eruptions of guttate psoriasis although a direct causal relationship has not been established. Furthermore, there is also evidence that these organisms can act as an on-going stimulus for the chronic form of the disease.

The current evidence for the involvement of streptococci in the pathogenesis of psoriasis is reviewed below.

5.1 Group A Streptococci as a Trigger for Guttate Psoriasis

Several authors have reported an association between acute guttate psoriasis (AGP), particularly in children and young adults, and a streptococcal throat infection at approximately 1–2 weeks before the onset of skin lesions.[1-4] GAS, and streptococcal groups C and G, produce streptolysin-O (see Sec. 5.4) and thus the measurement of the anti-streptolysin-O (ASO) titre has commonly been used to confirm recent streptococcal infections. In 1954, Norrlind reported that 18 out of 32 (56%) patients with AGP had raised ASO titres of 200 U/ml or more, and ten (31%) gave histories of an upper respiratory infection prior to the eruption.[1] In a further series of 65 patients with sudden, widespread guttate psoriasis, a preceding severe upper respiratory infection was present in 42 (66%) patients.

In another study of 20 patients with AGP, 17 (85%) had raised ASO titres, 11 (55%) gave a history of an acute upper respiratory infection preceding the AGP and 40% had both.[3]

When the haemolytic streptococci isolated from the throats of 200 patients with psoriasis were grouped according to the Lancefield classification, group A (*Streptococcus pyogenes*), the most pathogenic group, was present in 82% of guttate compared to 34% of CP psoriasis patients, 33% of which grew group B streptococci.[4] However, the presence of haemolytic streptococci in non-psoriatic controls was not investigated. In a later study, the frequency of GAS observed in AGP was much lower (26%) but increased compared to either CP psoriasis patients (14%) or controls (7%), whilst other haemolytic streptococci were found with equal frequency in the study and control populations.[5] This difference in reported frequencies of GAS infection in AGP may reflect an increased use of antibiotics by general practitioners prior to referral of these patients to the hospital dermatology clinic for diagnosis of skin lesions.

In addition, individual case reports have also implicated perianal skin infections by GAS in acute psoriatic eruptions.[6,7]

The serotypes of M protein, the major virulence factor and antigenic determinant of GAS (see Sec. 5.4.2), have not been widely studied in isolates from AGP patients. Two studies that were carried out both identified various M types, including those associated with rheumatic fever and glomerulonephritis,[5,8] but the types were the same as those prevalent in the community at the time.[5] It has been suggested that the unusual immunological response of patients with psoriasis to streptococcal infection affords protection from other more serious sequelae of streptococcal infection which rarely occur concomitantly with AGP.[9] Thus the evidence so far argues against the existence of "psoriasogenic" M serotypes.

Groups C and G haemolytic streptococci have also been isolated from the throat[4,8] and skin[10] of patients with guttate psoriasis. These groups of streptococci probably also possess type-specific, anti-phagocytic surface factors analogous to the M proteins of GAS.[11,12]

5.2 Group A Streptococci and CP Psoriasis

In addition to their role as precipitating factors for self-limiting acute psoriasis, haemolytic streptococci may also act as an on-going stimulus for the chronic form of the disease. Indeed, there have been several reports of elevated ASO titres[3,13] and/or positive GAS throat cultures[4,13] in a proportion of patients with CP psoriasis. Furthermore, treatment of patients with resistant, streptococcal-associated psoriasis (four of whom had CP psoriasis) with rifampicin combined with penicillin or erythromycin led to the substantial improvement or resolution of skin lesions suggesting that streptococcal antigens may be involved in persistent psoriasis.[14] In addition, streptococcal infection may also precipitate or exacerbate psoriatic arthritis[15] and the pustular form of psoriasis.[16]

5.3 Induction of Psoriatic Lesions by Streptococci

In 1945, while investigating the presence of bacterial allergy in dermatitis herpetiformis, Swartz noted that in some of the psoriatic patients used as controls, the intradermal injection of an autologous stool not only induced a psoriatic lesion at the site of injection, but also aggravated the pre-existing psoriasis.[17] It was subsequently established that the organism in the stool responsible for the effect was *Streptococcus faecalis*. Robinson obtained the same results when he repeated Swartz's experiments.[18] Indeed, the exacerbations of psoriasis induced by the injection of the *S. faecalis* vaccine were so severe in some patients that they had to withdraw from the study.

Similarly, a generalized eruption of pustular psoriasis was induced by the intradermal injection of 0.01 ml of *Streptococcus haemolyticus* in a patient from which GAS had been cultured from a pustule on the finger.[19] In a second report, intradermal testing produced a pustule at the site of an injection of 0.02 ml of *S. pyogenes* antigen in a patient with psoriasis.[20] This was associated with a fever, malaise, arthralagia of the knees and toes, as well as pharyngeal pain and dysphagia. A grossly inflammatory but non-pustular reaction developed at the site of a *S. viridans* antigen injection in the same patient, but none of the nine other commercially prepared bacterial antigens, including *S. faecalis*, produced an unusual local inflammatory response.[20] Furthermore, two out of ten patients with psoriasis vulgaris produced typical local scaling and a psoriatic papule approximately ten days after an intradermal injection of the *S. pyogenes* antigen. In contrast, ten normal controls showed no reaction, or a local erythema and oedema.[20]

It has been suggested that micro-organisms exert their effects in psoriasis via the Koebner reaction, and thus act as a non-specific form of trauma. This is however unlikely since the exacerbation of psoriasis at sites away from the trauma is rarely observed in non-microbial elicitation of the Koebner phenomemon.[21]

5.4 Streptococcal Antigens

5.4.1 *Extracellular Products*

GAS produce a variety of antigenic extracellular products, many of which have enzymatic and/or toxic activity. Antibodies against numerous different extracellular factors are found in human sera after GAS infections.

5.4.1.1 *Streptococcal pyrogenic exotoxins (SPEs)*

Three serologically distinct forms of streptococcal pyrogenic exotoxins (SPE-A, SPE-B and SPE-C), also known as erythrogenic or scarlet fever toxins, have been implicated not only in scarlet fever, but also in toxic shock-like syndrome, erysipelas and guttate psoriasis. These toxins possess several biological activities including pyrogenicity, skin reactivity, T cell stimulating activity and enhancement of host susceptibility to endotoxin lethality. However, their ability, in common with the enterotoxins produced by *Staphylococcus aureus* to act as potent T cell mitogens is probably their major mechanism of pathogenicity,[22] with the exception of SPE-B which has been identified as a proteinase precursor.[23]

The proportion of T cells in peripheral blood activated by these toxins is not, however, as large as that stimulated by plant lectins such as concanavalin A, but is much greater than that responding to an antigenic peptide. Investigation of the binding sites for toxins on the T cell receptor (TCR) led to an explanation for these differences in response. TCRs for antigenic peptides bound to MHC proteins are made up of five clonally variable components Vα, Jα, Vβ, Dβ and Jβ, as well as N region amino acids contributed by non-germline-encoded bases inserted at the junctions between Vα and Jα, Vβ and Dβ, and Dβ and Jβ. Recognition of conventional antigenic peptides bound to MHC proteins involves contributions from all the variable components of the TCR. In contrast, toxins stimulate T cells almost exclusively via the Vβ region of the TCR expressed by T cells.[24-26] Each toxin stimulates T cells bearing particular Vβ families which vary for each toxin (Table 5.1).

Furthermore, these so-called superantigens do not bind to those regions on the TCR believed to be involved in the binding of conventional antigenic peptide plus MHC, but instead bind to an exposed face of Vβ (Fig. 5.1). Plant lectins, on the other hand, bypass the TCR altogether and thus can stimulate all T cells regardless of the structure of their TCR.

Stimulation of T cells by toxins is dependent upon the presence of MHC Class II-positive cells in the cultures, but is not restricted by Class II alleles as is usually the case for antigenic peptides. The antigen-binding groove of MHC Class II molecules is formed between two polypeptide chains whose NH_2-terminal regions comprise an extended β-pleated sheet supporting two α helices. The foreign or self peptides normally lie in this cleft and are presented to T cells

Table 5.1 Vβ specificities of streptococcal superantigens

Superantigen	Vβ Specificity	Reference
SPE-A	8, 12, 14	24
	2, 12, 14, 15	25
	12	26
SPE-C	1, 2, 5.1, 10	25
SPE-F (MF)	2, 4, 8, 15, 19	28
	2, 7, 8, 18, 21	29
SPE-X	8	26
SSA	1, 3, 15	27
CAP	8	30
SPM-2	4, 7, 8	31

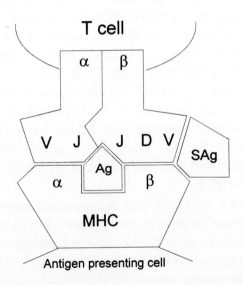

Fig. 5.1. Schematic representation of complex of MHC Class II, TCR and superantigen (SAg)/Antigen (Ag).

bearing TCR αβ receptors. However, the toxins bind outside of this groove.

Further superantigens synthesised by GAS have now been characterised. Streptococcal superantigen (SSA), whose amino terminus is more homologous to that of Staphylococcal enterotoxin-B, -C_1, and -C_3 (SEB, SEC_1, SEC_3) than those of SPE-A, SPE-B or SPE-C, activates human T cells expressing Vβ1, 3 or 15 (Table 5.1).[27] Streptococcal pyrogenic exotoxin F (SPE-F, previously referred to as mitogenic factor), whose gene could be detected in 42 GAS strains representing 14 serotypes, preferentially activated T cells bearing Vβ2, 4, 8, 15 and 19.[28] However, in a later study, T cells expressing Vβ2, 7, 8, 18 or 21 were shown to be selectively stimulated by this superantigen.[29] This variation in the findings, which was also a feature of investigations of the effects of SPE-A and SPE-C (Table 5.1), is probably related to the use of purified versus recombinant superantigens since purification is not always sufficiently rigorous to remove contaminating molecules.[26] In addition, a cytoplasmic-membrane-associated protein (CAP) has been isolated and shown to act as a superantigen.[30] A related molecule, *Streptococcus pyogenes* mitogen-2 (SPM-2), was isolated from the culture supernatant of *S. pyogenes* strain T12 but was not detected in the culture fluids of other streptococcal strains including groups B and D streptococci.[31]

5.4.1.2 *Streptococcal cytolytic toxins (haemolysins)*

The two streptococcal cytolysins have been designated streptolysin-S (produced in the presence of serum and is oxygen stable) and -O (oxygen labile and does not require serum for its production).[32]

Streptolysin-S is an unstable 32 amino acid polypeptide associated with various carrier molecules that both act as stabilizers and induce the release of the active haemolysin from its cell-bound state.[32] Streptolysin-S lyses a wide range of cells, both eukaryotic (it is largely responsible for the haemolysis seen on blood agar plates) and bacterial (protoplasts and L-forms which lack a cell wall). However, this haemolysin is apparently not immunogenic. The lack of induction of specific neutralising antibody may result from the suppression of T cell-dependent antibody responses by streptolysin-S or perhaps from the small size of the active polypeptide moiety.

In contrast, streptolysin-O is an antigenic protein with a Mwt of approximately 60,000, the quantitation of antibodies against which is a widely used means of diagnosis of recent GAS infections.[32] Streptolysin-O binds to cholesterol in the membranes of mammalian cells and induces their lysis. Its intense cardiotoxicity has suggested a role for this molecule in the pathogenesis of rheumatic fever and rheumatic heart disease. In contrast to patients with throat infections, patients with streptococcal impetigo or pyoderma often show weak or absent antibody responses to streptolysin-O (Table 5.2).[33,34]

5.4.1.3 Streptococcal enzymes

Other extracellular products of GAS that induce good humoral immune responses in man after an infection are nicotinamide-adenine-dinucleotide-glucohydrolase (NADase), streptokinase, hyaluronidase and the deoxyribonucleases (DNAses) (Table 5.2).[35]

NADase is a protein with a Mwt of approximately 55,000 which is produced predominately by nephritogenic streptococcal strains. Streptokinase (Mwt 47,600), which exists in at least two distinct antigenic entities, activates the fibrinolytic system of human blood via plasminogen. Hyaluronidase depolymerises hyaluronic acid on the mucous membrane of the oropharynx and may therefore encourage the spread of the organism within tissue.

The DNAses (Mwt 25-30,000) can be split into 4 antigenic types A, B, C and D. Nucleases A and C split DNA only whereas nucleases B and D split RNA as well. Increased levels of antibodies to DNAse B are observed in patients with GAS infections of the skin who produce low levels of ASO titres. Other extracellular products include the bacteriocins, lipoproteinases and other factors that have not yet been fully characterised.

Table 5.2   Immune response to extracellular products of group A streptococci

Protein	Humoral Response	T-Cell Mediated
Pyrogenic exotoxins: SPE-A, -B, -C, -F, -X	Yes deletion	Vβ-specific superantigens (except SPE-B): Proliferation, anergy,
Streptolysin-O	Increased with throat infection Decreased with skin infection (impetigo, pyoderma)	
Streptolysin-S	None	
NADase	Induced by nephritogenic strains	
Streptokinase (two antigenic types)	Yes	Proliferation (MHC-Class II-restricted) Hypersensitivity reactions
Hyaluronidase	Increased with skin infection	
DNase (A, B, C, D)	DNase B antibs increased in skin infection	

5.4.2 *Cellular Proteins*

Numerous different proteins are found on the cell wall and membrane of GAS. Considerable progress has been made in identifying and characterising several of the cell wall proteins including the M protein, receptors for IgG and IgA and T protein. In contrast, little is known about the proteins present on the streptococcal membrane with the exception of the anchor region of the M protein, which includes a highly conserved sequence of amino acids found at the C-terminus of different proteins expressed by various organisms.

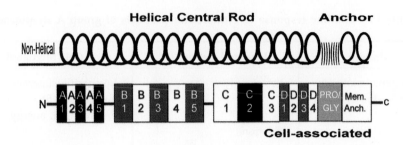

Fig. 5.2. Structure of M6 molecule consisting of blocks of repeated amino acid sequences (A, B, C, D), a region rich in proline and glycine that crosses the cell wall, and amino acids at the C-terminus that allow attachment to the cell membrane.

5.4.2.1 *M and M-like proteins*

The M protein is the major virulence factor and type-specific antigen of GAS. It is an α-helical coiled coil on the surface of the organism consisting of a variable N-terminal half and a C-terminus which is conserved between serotypes which now number more than 80.[36] Approximately 80% of the M6 molecule (which is representative of the M protein family) is made up of 4 distinct regions (A–D), each of which consists of repeated sequences of amino acids (Fig. 5.2).[36]

Region A, together with a 11 amino acid non-helical sequence at the N-terminus of the molecule farthest from the bacterial cell, form a hypervariable region which is the target for neutralising antibodies. Only antibodies specific for this region permit phagocytes to engulf the streptococci. Adjacent to region D at the C-terminal end is a non-repeat region containing predominately proline and glycine amino acids which passes through the cell wall. Next to that is a region of hydrophobic amino acids which form an anchor in the membrane. A short six amino acid sequence (LPSTGE) adjacent to the hydrophobic region is highly conserved in all the known surface proteins of gram-positive bacteria. This region has proved to be essential for the attachment of the M protein to the organism.[37]

M proteins share as much as 40% amino acid identity with other fibrous coiled coil proteins such as tropomyosin,[38] myosin[39] and keratin.[40] In addition, cross-reactivity of M protein with antigens including those in the synovium[41] and brain,[42] as well as heat shock proteins[43] have also been demonstrated.

Other surface proteins with affinity for IgG and/or IgA have, more recently, been isolated and characterised from different strains of *S. pyogenes*.[44,45] These proteins have extensive amino acid sequence similarities to M protein in the proline-rich region, membrane anchor sequence and cytoplasmic domain.[46] Indeed the genes coding for M proteins and these M-like Fc receptor proteins are considered to be products of gene duplication.[46] However, in contrast to M proteins, immunoglobulin-binding streptococcal proteins have not been shown to play a role in pathogenicity or virulence (Table 5.3). Similarly, trypsin-resistant T protein, another streptococcal surface protein with amino acid sequence similarities to M protein in the C-terminal region,[47] does not enhance virulence or induce protective antibody.

5.4.2.2 *Other cell wall proteins*

The initial adherence of *S. pyogenes* to epithelial cells of the upper respiratory tract is thought to involve its ability to bind fibronectin which is mediated by the fibronectin receptor, protein F, and by various other streptococcal ligands found on the surface of the bacterium (Table 5.3).[48,49] In addition, glyceraldehyde-3-phosphate-dehydrogenase, a further major surface protein of group A streptococci, has been shown to have both enzymatic activity and a binding capacity for a variety of proteins such as fibronectin, lysozyme, actin and myosin.[50]

A protein with C5a peptidase activity is also present on the bacterial surface.[51] Furthermore, the gene encoding a 67 kDa surface protein with no significant similarity to any known streptococcal protein has been cloned and sequenced.[52] Despite its different structure, this protein was cross-reactive with myosin suggesting that anti-myosin antibodies recognised conformational epitopes common to both proteins. This protein also exhibited a significant amount of identity

Table 5.3 Streptococcal cell surface proteins

Protein	Streptococcal Group	Similarity to M Protein	Binds to	Trypsin-sensitivity
M specific)	A, C, G (type- Fibronectin	— Fibrinogen,	Albumin, IgG,	S
IgG/IgA FcR	A	C-terminal Pro/gly & Anchor regions	Albumin, IgG/IgA	ND
T type-specific)	A (limited	As above	Fibrinogen	R
F FBP S4	A A	ND Lacks LPXTG Fibrinogen	Fibronectin, LCs Fibronectin,	S S
Glyc-3-P-Dehydrog	A, B, C, E, G, L	None Actin	Fibronectin, Lysozyme, Myosin,	S
C5a peptidase	A, G	None	C5a	R
67 kD Ag	A. G	None	ND	ND

ND = Not done; S = trypsin-sensitive; R = trypsin-resistant.

and similarity to the β chain of Class II MHC molecules of mice and humans.

5.4.2.3 *Membrane proteins*

Information relating to the identity of proteins present on the streptococcal membrane is, in contrast, limited. SDS-PAGE analysis of GAS membranes revealed a minimum of 60 polypeptides, four of which (Mwts 22–32 kDa) were identified as constituting an antigen cross-reactive with sarcolemmal sheaths of cardiac myofibres.[53] Furthermore, the 67 kDa myosin cross-reactive cell wall protein also appears to be present in the membrane; membrane antigenic determinants shared with glomerular basement membrane have also been described.

5.5 Immune Response to Extracellular Streptococcal Proteins and Superantigens

5.5.1 *Humoral Response*

As described earlier, ASO titres have been reported to be raised in at least half of patients with guttate psoriasis[1,2] compared to 12% in normal subjects. Based upon a significant association between HLA-A13 and a history of severe streptococcal infection in psoriasis, Bertrams *et al.*[54] measured ASO titres in 110 patients with psoriasis who were typed for HLA-A13 antigen. Surprisingly, ASO titres were significantly decreased in the HLA-A13[+] compared to HLA-A13[-] group. However, no information was given as to whether the HLA-A13[+] patients in the study had guttate or CP psoriasis, or whether they had a history of streptococcal infections.

Evidence of streptococcal infections in psoriasis patients has also been established by measurement of antibodies to deoxyribonuclease B and hyaluronidase, two other extracellular products of streptococci.[5,55] Furthermore, levels of anti-DNAse B antibodies have been shown to be raised in psoriatic arthritis patients compared to patients with psoriasis without arthritis, rheumatoid arthritis, other forms of dermatitis and normal controls.[15]

Recently, immunoblotting has been used to study the humoral response of 26 patients with acute guttate psoriasis to soluble antigens derived from streptococci which had been frozen, repeatedly disrupted and then centrifuged to remove cell debris.[56] Eighteen patients had a demonstrable response to a wide range of streptococcal antigens using this approach whilst only 14 has raised ASO titres. Although the bands were heavier and more numerous than for the controls, there did not appear to be any antibody protein bands specific for guttate psoriasis. Furthermore, antibody responses were observed to streptococci of groups C and G as well as of group A suggesting recognition of antigens common to the three Lancefield groups.

In contrast, antibodies to CAP/SCAP superantigen were not significantly different in moderately to severely affected psoriatic patients compared to those of healthy controls.[57]

5.5.2 *In Vivo/In Vitro Response to SK/SD*

When normal and psoriatic individuals were skin tested with Dermatophytin-O, tuberculin purified protein derivative (PPD) and the GAS extracellular enzymes streptokinase/streptodornase (SK/SD), the latter showed a significant decrease in the amount (but not incidence) of both erythema and induration to SK/SD.[58] However, there was no correlation between this altered cell-mediated response to SK/SD and the extent or activity of the psoriatic skin lesions in individual patients. Similar results have been reported in two earlier studies.[59,60] Furthermore, a delay in the resolution of the delayed hypersensitivity reaction to SK/SD, compared to non-psoriatic controls, was observed in a group of 12 psoriasis patients who were examined for up to 28 days after intradermal injection for the development of psoriasis.[61] However, SK/SD was not able to induce a positive Koebner reaction in these patients under the conditions used in the study.

In contrast, the *in vitro* PBL proliferative response by psoriatic patients to SK/SD was markedly higher than that of non-psoriatic individuals, but this difference did not reach statistical significance.[62]

5.5.3 *Superantigens*

Although an increased *in vitro* proliferative response to the staphylococcal superantigens SEB and TSST-1 was observed in blood and/or skin,[63,64] PBL from psoriatic patients were shown to be hyporesponsive to the streptococcal superantigen CAP/SCAP.[57] This decrease in response was only partially explained by the presence of specific inhibitors in the serum; a lower affinity or alteration in binding of psoriatic MHC Class II to the superantigen may be responsible.

The first indication that superantigens may be important in the pathogenesis of psoriasis came from the finding that Vβ2$^+$, and to a lesser extent Vβ5.1$^+$ T lymphocytes, were markedly overexpressed in the skin of patients with guttate and CP psoriasis.[65] The streptococcal toxins, SPE-A, SPE-C and SPE-F stimulate T cells expressing Vβ2; SPE-C also stimulates Vβ5.1$^+$ T cells (Table 5.1). In addition, the N-terminal half of M5 protein cleaved by pepsin (pep M5) has also been shown to act as a superantigen activating Vβ2$^+$ (Vβ4$^+$ and Vβ8$^+$) T cells.[66] However, it has been suggested subsequently that the latter's effects are probably mediated by contaminating extoxins.[67]

Confirmation of the expansion of Vβ2$^+$ T cells in acute guttate psoriatic skin followed, together with sequence analysis of the TCR Vβ2$^+$ genes which revealed extensive junctional region diversity compatible with a superantigen rather than a conventional antigen-driven T cell response.[68] In support of this idea, all streptococcal isolates from the patients in the study were shown to secrete SPE-C. Exacerbation of CP psoriasis by superantigens produced by *S. aureus* and *C. albicans* have also been reported.[69]

The selective homing of T cells to the skin in humans has been shown to involve the interaction of the oligosaccharide epitope CLA on T cells with E-selectin expressed by endothelial cells.[70,71] Recently, it has been demonstrated that bacterial superantigens (both staphylococcal and streptococcal toxins) induce the expansion of skin-homing CLA$^+$ T cells via stimulation of IL-12 production.[72] Thus, streptococcal exotoxins may contribute to the psoriatic process both by activation of T cells and by inducing their homing to the skin.

5.6 Immune Response to Streptococcal Cellular Proteins

5.6.1 *Streptococcal Cell Walls and Membranes*

PBMC responses to group A streptococcal antigens (cell wall, cell membranes or sonicated whole cells) are significantly increased in patients with guttate and CP psoriasis using a 2-step leukocyte migration inhibition agarose test[73] or proliferation assay,[74] respectively (Fig. 5.3).

Furthermore, the PBL proliferative response to sonicated whole cell type M22 streptococci was significantly reduced after repeated

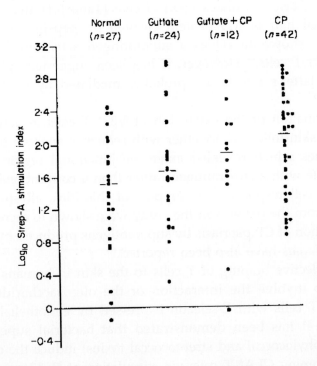

Fig. 5.3. Proliferative PBMC responses to sonicated GAS (Strep-A) in patients with guttate, CP, or guttate plus CP psoriasis compared to normal controls. (Source: Baker B.S. *et al. Br.J.Dermatol.* **125** (1991), 38–42, with permission from Blackwell Science Ltd, Oxford, UK.)

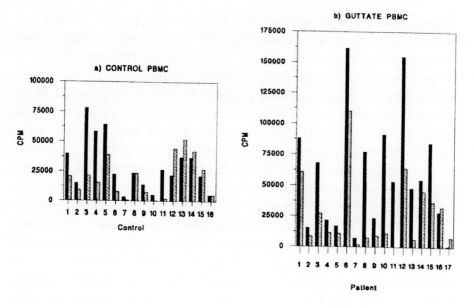

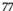

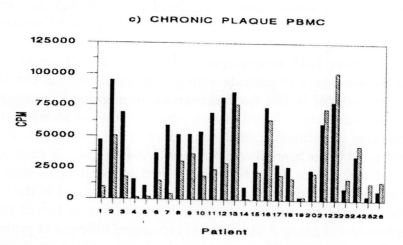

Fig. 5.4. Proliferative response of PBMC from (a) non-psoriatic controls, (b) guttate and (c) CP patients to Strep M22 and Strep-M22T (Strep-M22 trypsinized to remove M protein) ■ Strep-M22 ▨ Strep-M22T. (Source: Baker B.S. *et al. Acta Dermatol.Venereol. (Stockh)* **74** (1994), 276–278, with permission from Scandinavian University Press, Oslo, Norway.)

trypsinization in both guttate and CP psoriasis patient groups but not in that of normal controls (Fig. 5.4).[75] These results suggest that there is an increased frequency of T lymphocytes specific for a trypsin-sensitive streptococcal protein (possibly M22 or M-like protein) in the blood of these patients. However, trypsinized M22-streptococci were still able to induce substantial proliferation of psoriatic (and normal) PBL indicating that T cells reactive with trypsin-resistant streptococcal proteins were also present.

In contrast, decreased PBL proliferative responses to a potent immunopotentiator OK-432, a preparation of penicillin-treated, low virulence Su-strain of *S. pyogenes* group A3, has also been reported in psoriasis.[76] This preparation has been widely used for cancer therapy and exerts its anti-tumour effects by augmentation of macrophage cytotoxicity and natural killer cell activity, and induction of HLA-DR on monocytes through the production of various cytokines such as IFN-γ and TNF-α. The authors suggest that their findings may reflect an abnormality at the level of T cell and monocyte interaction, but this explanation is not consistent with the increased response to group A streptococcal antigens as described above.

In addition, GAS antigen-specific TCL have been isolated from skin lesions from 5/5 patients with guttate psoriasis.[77] In contrast, only seven out of 18 TCL isolated from a control group (consisting of patients with eczema, lichen planus, pityriasis rosea or nickel contact dermatitis, and three normal individuals skin tested with PPD) proliferated to the heat-killed isolates of GAS (see Chap. 3, Table 3.2). One of the guttate TCL (NY) was cloned by limiting dilution in the presence of type five streptococcal M protein. Eight of the nine clones isolated reacted, to a varying extent, to one or two of three preparations of group A streptococci expressing different M proteins (see Chap. 3, Fig. 3.4). The streptococcal response of four consistently reactive clones from this patient was HLA-DR restricted (Table 5.4) and inhibited by anti-HLA-DR antibody in a dose-dependent manner. On stimulation, these four clones secreted high levels of IFN-γ and detectable levels of IL-2, IL-10 and GM-CSF, but no IL-4 or TNF-α production was detected (Fig. 5.5).

Table 5.4 HLA-DR restriction of the Strep-A1-specific proliferative responses of clones NY 5, 7, 8 and 9. (Source: Baker B.S. *et al. Br.J.Dermatol.* 128 (1993), 493–499, with permission from Blackwell Science Ltd, Oxford, UK.)

Clone	Antigen Presenting Cells			
	DR 4, 8	DR 5(11)[†]	DR 4, w13	DR 5(11), 8*
NY 5	16,171 (1,945)	NR	NR	25,223 (2,917)
NY 7	25,136 (1,719)	NR	NR	32,882 (1,912)
NY 8	39,059 (3,339)	NR	NR	49,161 (6,830)
NY 9	5,986 (386)	NR	NR	8,625 (351)

Data are expressed as mean c.p.m. of clone in the presence of Strep-A1 minus clone in the absence of Strep-A1. (Background counts of clones in the absence of antigen ranged from 77 to 1,704 c.p.m.) Standard deviations are shown in parentheses. NR, no response (defined as < 1,000 c.p.m.) *Autologous PBMC from patient NY. [†]EBV B-cell line.

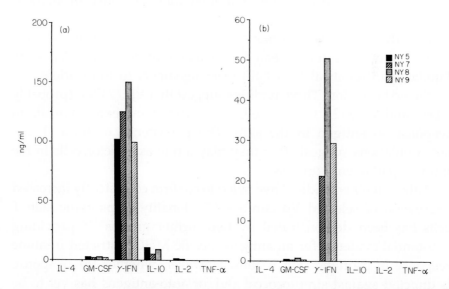

Fig. 5.5. Cytokine production by Con A (a) and anti-CD3 plus PMA (b)-stimulated NY skin T cell clones. (Source: Baker B.S. *et al. Br.J.Dermatol.* **128** (1993), 493–499, with permission from Blackwell Science Ltd, Oxford, UK.)

Furthermore, streptococcal antigen-specific TCL have also been isolated from CP lesions from 64% of the patients (16 out of 25) studied.[78] The majority of this patient group had no serological evidence of a recent infection.

Further evidence for an antigen-specific (rather than super-antigenic) immune response has come from Vβ TCR analysis of CP lesions.[79,80] Overexpression of either or both Vβ2 and Vβ6 gene families were demonstrated in a study which characterized the TCR repertoires of normal and psoriatic skin lesions. However, sequence analysis of the CDR3 of these Vβ gene families showed a marked oligoclonality only in psoriatic lesions, but not in normal skin or psoriatic PBL.[79]

In contrast, increased expression of the Vβ3 and/or Vβ13.1 gene families was demonstrated when T cells were isolated from the epidermis of CP lesions and separated into CD4+ and CD8+ T cell subsets.[80] Only the CD8+ T cell subset showed this preferential TCR expression and, furthermore, exhibited monoclonality or marked oligoclonality.[80]

In both studies, second biopsies taken from some of the patients several months later revealed expansion of the same Vβ gene families and identical Vβ CDR3 rearrangements to those identified on the first occasion. These findings suggest that Vβ2+/Vβ6+ (probably CD4+) and Vβ3/13.1 CD8+ T cells are recruited and expand *in situ* in response to antigen in the skin. The persistence of these T cell subpopulations suggests that they play a role as effector cells in the immunopathogenic process.

Although other studies have failed to confirm consistently increased expression of selected Vβ families,[81,82] clonality of psoriatic skin T cells has been demonstrated by two further groups[83,84] providing substantial evidence for an antigen-specific MHC-restricted immune response in psoriatic skin lesions. However, whether this response is directed against streptococcal and/or auto-antigens has yet to be determined.

5.6.2 *Streptococcal M Protein*

It has been shown that T cells in lesional skin of patients with guttate or CP psoriasis can recognise sonicated, heat-killed group A streptococci of more than one M serotype. The next question to be addressed was, therefore, the identity of the streptococcal antigen(s) involved. The most likely candidate appeared to be the M protein since it is the major antigenic determinant of the organism. Furthermore, since the response was not restricted to any particular M serotype, the conserved C-terminal rather than the variable N-terminal half was implicated. Homology between M protein and keratin involving the heptapeptide repeat patterns which form the alpha-helical coiled-coil structure in both molecules has been demonstrated suggesting that cross-reactive T cells specific for both M protein and a skin autoantigen may be relevant to the disease process.[85]

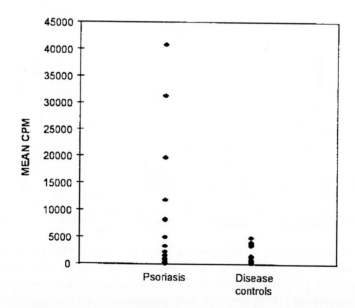

Fig. 5.6. Proliferative response by PBMC from CP psoriatic versus disease control patients to rM6.

Studies carried out to demonstrate T cell recognition of M protein in psoriasis have, however, produced mixed findings. Thus, as mentioned above (Sec. 5.6.1), an increased frequency of peripheral blood T cells specific for a trypsin-sensitive streptococcal protein has been reported in guttate and CP psoriatic patients.[75] However, it should be noted that M and M-like proteins are not the only surface proteins expressed by group A streptococci that are sensitive to digestion by trypsin (Table 5.3). Futhermore, when PBMC from psoriatic patients were tested with purified recombinant M6 protein, variable proliferative responses were observed (Fig. 5.6). The majority of patients showed weak responses and overall these did not differ from that of disease controls.

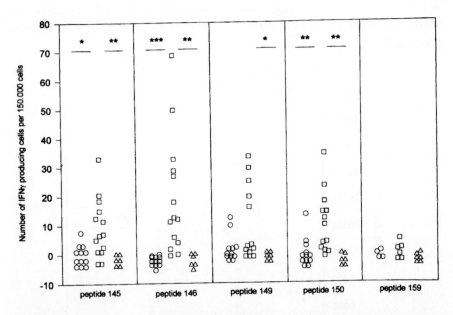

Fig. 5.7. T cell responses to M6 peptides 145, 146, 149 and 150 sharing sequences with keratins, and control peptide 159, as evaluated by ELISPOT. f Healthy controls, ○ patients with psoriasis, or Δ atopic dermatitis. (Source: Sigmundsdottir H. *et al. Scand.J.Immunol.* **45** (1997), 688–697, with permission from Blackwell Science Ltd, Oxford, UK.)

In contrast, significantly increased IFN-γ production in response to three M6-peptides sharing sequences with type I keratins was demonstrated in untreated psoriasis patients compared to paired healthy controls (Fig. 5.7).[86] Patients with atopic dermatitis did not respond to any of the M6 peptides, and IFN-γ response to a control M6-peptide which did not share sequences with keratins was negligible in all groups. Furthermore, the IFN-γ response to all the M6-peptides, but not to SK/SD, was almost abolished after successful treatment of the psoriatic skin lesions suggesting that the presence of circulating TH$_1$ cells specific for M6-peptides may precede or coincide with the appearance of psoriatic lesions.

However, because only five or six of the 20 amino acids constituting the M6-peptides from the C-terminal region of M protein were shared with type I keratins, it would be premature to conclude that the T cell epitope recognised by psoriatic T cells in each case encompasses these shared amino acids. In addition, part of these M6 sequences are also shared by another molecule of similar structure, myosin. Thus the significance of the restricted homology with keratin exhibited by these M6-peptides to the increased psoriatic response remains to be demonstrated.

In psoriatic skin, investigations of M protein reactivity of T cells have also produced conflicting results. Thus, GAS-reactive TCL isolated from CP psoriatic lesions show a significantly decreased response to cell wall extract from a M negative mutant (whose gene encoding for M protein had been deleted) compared to that of the corresponding M6-expressing streptococci, hence suggesting M protein recognition (Fig. 5.8) (Baker B.S. *et al.*, unpublished observations). However, only approximately half of the TCL responded to the M6-positive cell wall extract, and none of them proliferated in response to purified recombinant M6 protein. The lack of response to the latter may, however, be explained by differences in antigen processing of the recombinant M protein.

Interestingly, when GAS-reactive TCL from guttate psoriatic lesions were tested with trypsinized streptococci, in contrast to PBL (Fig. 5.4), a doubling of response was observed in some cases compared to that

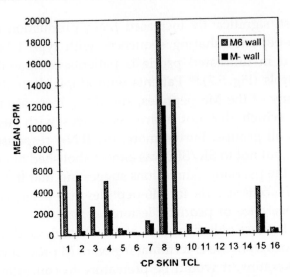

Fig. 5.8. Response to M6 versus M-neg cell wall extracts by GAS-reactive TCL from CP psoriatic lesions.

Table 5.5   Differential proliferative response by guttate skin TCL to trypsinized (A1T, A2T) versus untrypsinized (A1, A2) GAS

TCL	A1	A1T	A2	A2T	MED
1	525	1,319	4,549	669	282
2	24,440	**43,410**	35,135	44,066	2,953
3	4,917	5,180	11,937	**21,316**	158
4	2,325	1,424	16,664	2,737	145
5	38,097	37,238	45,155	16,806	73
6	18,867	**41,821**	1,041	**46,383**	107
7	1,729	**6,084**			1,995
8	261	**1,994**			32

Data are given in mean cpm; bold type indicates marked increase in response to trypsinized versus untrypsinized. A1 and A2 are M22- and M1-expressing GAS, which after repeated trypsinization to remove M-like proteins, are designated A1T and A2T, respectively. MED denotes culture in medium without antigen.

of the untrypsinized bacteria. (Table 5.5) (Baker B.S. *et al.,* unpublished observations.) This suggested recognition of a molecule(s) unmasked by the removal of M and M-like molecules.

The above findings suggest that GAS-reactive TCL from psoriatic skin lesions may contain a mixture of T cells which recognise M and non-M cell wall proteins.

5.6.3 *Streptococcal Membrane Proteins*

A recent study has shown that the responses induced by proteins from the M6 streptococcal membrane are significantly higher than those induced by M6 cell wall proteins, both for PBMC and GAS-reactive TCL isolated from skin lesions of CP psoriatic patients (Fig. 5.9) (Baker B.S. *et al.,* unpublished observations.) The identity of the membrane protein(s) that induce the T cell response are unknown and the subject of current investigation.

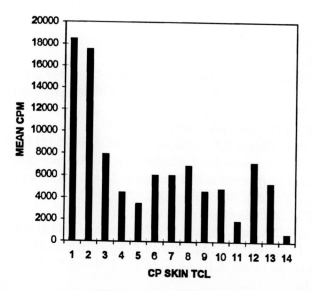

Fig. 5.9. Response to streptococcal M6 membrane extract by GAS-reactive TCL from CP skin lesions.

5.6.4 *CLA Induction by Group A Streptococcal Antigens*

In common with bacterial toxins, GAS antigens have been shown to induce CLA expression by T cells in an IL-12-dependent manner.[87] In patients with psoriasis, but not in controls, streptococcal antigens modulate specific tissue-homing receptors on T cells in a differential manner inducing significantly higher CLA[+] T cell numbers than *C. albicans* whilst down-regulating T cell expression of the peripheral lymph node-selective homing receptor, L-selectin.[87] These effects on homing receptor T cell expression would favour increased selective migration into the skin of streptococcal antigen-specific T cells. Thus, susceptibility of psoriatic patients to develop skin lesions subsequent to a GAS infection may, in part, be due to this altered response by psoriatic T cells to streptococcal antigen-induced homing receptors.

References

1. Norrlind R. *Acta Rheum.Scand.* **1** (1955), 135–144.
2. Whyte H.J. and Baughman R.D. *Arch.Dermatol.* **89** (1964), 350–356.
3. Norholm-Pedersen A. *Acta Dermatol.Venereol. (Stockh)* **32** (1952), 159–164.
4. Cohen-Tervaert W.C., Esseveld H. *Dermatologica* **140** (1970), 282–290.
5. Telfer N.R., Chalmers R.J.G., Whale K., Colman G. *Arch.Dermatol.* **128** (1992), 39–42.
6. Honig P.J. *J.Paediatr.* **113** (1988), 1037–1039.
7. Rehder P.A., Eliezer E.T., Lane A.T. *Arch.Dermatol.* **124** (1988), 702–704.
8. Belew P.W., Wannamaker L.W., Johnson D., Rosenberg E.W. In *Recent Advances in Streptococci and Streptococcal Diseases*, Kimura K., Kotami S., Shiokawa Y. (eds), Reedbooks Ltd., UK (1985), p. 334.
9. Belew P.W. *Arch.Dermatol.* **119** (1983), 3.
10. Henderson C.A. and Highet A.S. *Br.J.Dermatol.* **118** (1988), 559–562.
11. Bisno A.L., Craven D.E., McCabe W.R. *Infect.Immun.* **55** (1987), 753–757.
12. Efstratiou A., Teare E.L., McGhie D., Colman G. *J.Infect.* **19** (1989), 105–111.
13. Haro H.S., Patiala R., Widholm O. *Ann. Med. Intern.* **43** (1954), 216–225.
14. Rosenberg E.W. *et al. J.Am.Acad.Dermatol.* **14** (1986), 761–764.

15. Vasey B. *et al. J.Rheumatol.* **9** (1982), 719–722.
16. Baker H. and Ryan T.J. *Br.J.Dermatol.* **80** (1968), 771–793.
17. Swartz J.H. *N.Engl.J.Med.* **233** (1945), 296–297.
18. Robinson M.M. *J.Invest.Dermatol.* **20** (1953), 455–459.
19. Landry M. and Muller S.A. *Arch.Dermatol.* **105** (1972), 711–716.
20. Shelley W.B., Gray Wood M., Beerman H. *J.Invest.Dermatol.* **65** (1975), 466–471.
21. Rosenberg E.W. and Noah P.W. *J.Am.Acad.Dermatol.* **18** (1988), 151–158.
22. Gerlach D. *et al. Zbl.Bakteriol.Hyg.A.* **255** (1983), 221–233.
23. Marrack P. and Kappler J. *Science* **248** (1990), 705–711.
24. Abe J. *et al. J.Immunol.* **146** (1991), 3747–3750.
25. Tomai M.A., Schlievert P.M., Kotb M. *Infect.Immun.* **60** (1992), 701–705.
26. Braun M.A. *et al. J.Immunol.* **150** (1993), 2457–2465.
27. Mollick J.A. *et al. J.Clin.Invest.* **92** (1993), 710–719.
28. Norrby-Teglund A. *et al. Infect.Immun.* **62** (1994), 5227–5233.
29. Toyosaki T. *et al. Eur.J.Immunol.* **26** (1996), 2693–2701.
30. Sato H., Itoh T., Rikiishi H., Kumagai K. *Microbiol.Immunol.* **38** (1994), 139–147.
31. Rikiishi H. *et al. Immunol.* **91** (1997), 406–413.
32. Wannamaker L.W. *Reviews Infect.Dis.* **5, Suppl.** 4 (1983), 5723–5732.
33. Wannamaker L.W. *N.Engl.J.Med.* **282** (1970), 23–31.
34. Wannamaker L.W. *N.Engl.J.Med.* **282** (1970), 78–85.
35. Stollerman G.H. In *Streptococci and Streptococcal Diseases*, Wannamaker L.W. and Matsen J.M. (eds), Academic, New York (1972).
36. Phillips G.N. *et al. Proc.Natl.Acad.Sci. (USA)* **78** (1981), 4689–4693.
37. Schneewind O., Pancholi V., Fischetti V.A. In *New Perspectives on Streptococci and Streptococcal Infections, Zbl.Bakt.*, Orefici G. (ed), Gustav Fischer, Stuttgart, **Suppl.** 22 (1992), 174–176.
38. Fenderson P.G., Fischetti V.A., Cunningham M.W. *J.Immunol.* **142** (1989), 2475–2481.
39. Dale J.B. and Beachey E.H. *J.Exp.Med.* **162** (1985), 583–591.
40. Swerlick R.A., Cunningham M.W., Hall N.K. *J.Invest.Dermatol.* **87** (1986), 367–371.
41. Baird R.W. *et al. J.Immunol.* **146** (1991), 3132–3137.
42. Bronze M.S. and Dale J.B. *J.Immunol.* **151** (1993), 2820–2828.
43. Quinn A., Shinnick T.M., Cunningham M.W. *Infect.Immun.* **64** (1996), 818–824.

44. Heath D.G. and Cleary P.P. *Infect.Immun.* **55** (1987), 1232–1238.
45. Gomi H. *et al. J.Immunol.* **144** (1990), 4046–4052.
46. Heath D.G. and Cleary P.P. *Proc.Natl.Acad.Sci. (USA)* **86** (1989), 4741–4745.
47. Schneewind O., Jones K.F., Vischetti V.A. *J.Bacteriol.* **172** (1990), 3310–3317.
48. Hanski E. and Caparon M.G. *Proc.Natl.Acad.Sci. (USA)* **89** (1992), 6172–6176.
49. Courtney H.S., Li Y., Dale J.B., Hasty D.L. *Infect.Immun.* **62** (1994), 3937–3946.
50. Pancholi V. and Fischetti V.A. *J.Exp.Med.* **176** (1992), 415–426.
51. Wexler D.E., Chenoweth E.E., Cleary P.P. *Proc. Natl.Acad.Sci. (USA)* **82** (1985), 8144–8148.
52. Kil K.S., Cunningham M.W., Barnett L.A. *Infect.Immun.* **62** (1994), 2440–2449.
53. Van de Rijn I., Zabriskie J.B., McCarty M. *J.Exp.Med.* **146** (1977), 579–599.
54. Bertrams J., Lattke C.L., Kuwert E. *N.Engl.J.Med.* **291** (1974), 631.
55. Quimby S.R., Markowitz H., Winkelman R.K. *Acta Dermatol.Venereol. (Stockh)* **60** (1980), 485–490.
56. Wilson A.G.McT. *et al. Br.J.Dermatol.* **128** (1993), 151–158.
57. Horiuchi N. *et al. Br.J.Dermatol.* **138** (1998), 229–235.
58. Krueger G.G., Hill H.R., Jederberg W.W. *J.Invest.Dermatol.* **71** (1978), 189–194.
59. Landau J.W. *et al. Arch.Dermatol.* **91** (1965), 607–611.
60. Rimbaud P. *et al. Bull Soc.Franc.Dermatol.Syphil.* **1** (1973), 477–478.
61. McFadden J.P. *et al. Acta Dermatol.Venereol. (Stockh)* **70** (1989), 262–264.
62. Baker B.S. *et al. Br.J.Dermatol.* **125** (1991), 38–42.
63. Yokote R., Tokura Y., Furukawa F., Takigawa M. *Arch.Dermatol.Res.* **287** (1995), 443–447.
64. Bour H. *et al. Acta Dermatol.Venereol. (Stockh)* **75** (1995), 218–221.
65. Lewis H. *et al. Br.J.Dermatol.* **129** (1993), 514–520.
66. Tomai M., Kotb M., Majumdar G., Beachey E.H. *J.Exp.Med.* **172** (1990), 359–362.
67. Fleischer B., Schmidt K.H., Gerlach D., Kohler W. *Infect.Immun.* **60** (1992), 1767–1770.
68. Leung D.Y.M. *et al. J.Clin.Invest.* **96** (1995), 2106–2112.

69. Leung D.Y.M., Walsh P., Giorno R., Norris D.A. *J.Invest.Dermatol.* **100** (1993), 225–228.
70. Picker L.J., Michie S.A., Rott L.S., Butcher E.C. *Am.J.Pathol.* **136** (1990), 1053–1068.
71. Picker L.J. *et al. Nature (London)* **349** (1991), 796–811.
72. Leung D.Y.M. *et al. J.Exp.Med.* **181** (1995), 747–753.
73. Gross W.L. *et al. Br.J.Dermatol.* **97** (1977), 529–537.
74. Baker B.S. *et al. Br.J.Dermatol.* **125** (1991), 38–42.
75. Baker B.S. *et al. Acta Dermatol.Venereol. (Stockh)* **74** (1994), 276–278.
76. Aiba S. and Tagami H. *Arch.Dermatol.Res.* **281** (1989), 310–315.
77. Baker B.S. *et al. Br.J.Dermatol.* **128** (1993), 493–499.
78. Baker B.S. *et al. Arch.Dermatol.Res.* **291** (1999), 564–566.
79. Menssen A. *et al. J.Immunol.* **155** (1995), 4078–4083.
80. Chang J.C.C. *et al. Proc.Natl.Acad.Sci. (USA)* **91** (1994), 9282–9286.
81. Boehncke W.H. *et al. J.Invest.Dermatol.* **104** (1995), 725–728.
82. Vekony M.A. *et al. J.Invest.Dermatol.* **109** (1997), 5–13.
83. Ahangari G. *et al. Scand.J.Immunol.* **45** (1997), 534–540.
84. Prinz J.C. *et al. Eur.J.Immunol.* **29** (1999), 3360–3368.
85. McFadden J.P., Valdimarsson H., Fry L. *Br.J.Dermatol.* **125** (1991), 443–447.
86. Sigmundsdottir H. *et al. Scand.J.Immunol.* **45** (1997), 688–697.
87. Baker B.S. *et al. Arch.Dermatol.Res.* **289** (1997), 671–676.

CHAPTER 6

Immune Function of Psoriatic Keratinocytes

It has become increasingly evident over the last decade that keratinocytes (KC) function as immunocompetent cells and should therefore be regarded as part of the skin immune system.

Thus, KC, in response to a variety of stimuli, are capable of producing a large number of proinflammatory and immuno-modulatory cytokines. In addition, they can respond to many of these cytokines in an autocrine manner via specific receptors on their surface. Upon activation, KC are able to express a variety of cell surface markers that are thought to be involved in antigen presentation and interaction with other cell types, particularly LCs and T cells.

6.1 Cytokine Production

KC are able to produce many of the same cytokines synthesized by T cells, with the exception of IL-2 and IFN-γ, and in addition produce EGF/TGF-α which is specifically produced by epithelial cells.

In psoriasis, several cytokines show altered expression including IL-1, IL-6, IL-8, IFN-γ and TGF-α (Table 6.1). Each cytokine will be discussed individually, although these cytokines undoubtedly do not act in isolation *in vivo* but interact with each other to produce functional effects.

Table 6.1   Altered expression of cytokines and growth factors and their receptors in psoriatic KC

Cytokine	Incr/Decr	Cytok.R/Inhib	Incr/Decr	Inducers
IL-1α	Decr	IL-1RI	Normal	Injury, LPS, UV light
IL-1β	Incr	IL-1RII IL-Ira	Incr Incr	IL-1, TNF-α, IFN-γ
IL-6	Incr	IL-6R	ND	LPS, UV, toxins, IL-1, IL-6, IFN-γ, TGF-β, TNF-α, viruses
IL-7	Incr	IL-7R	ND	IFN-γ
IL-8	Incr	IL-8R	Incr	LPS, IL-1, TNF-α IFN-γ
gro-α	Incr			
IP-10	Incr			IFN-γ
IL-10	Incr	IL-10R	Decr	UV, tape stripping, DTH
MCP-1/MCAF	Incr in basal KC			IL-1, TNF-α, IFN-γ
IL-12	Incr	IL-12R	ND	Bacteria, bacterial products
TNF-α	Incr	TNFR1	Normal	LPS, UV, IL-1, IL-2, IL-6, GMCSF, IFN-γ
		TNFR2	Absent	
Growth Factor	**Incr/Decr**	**Growth Fact.R**	**Incr/Decr**	**Inducers**
TGF-α/EGF	Incr	EGFR	Incr	TGF-α, IFN-γ
AG	Incr	EGFR	Incr	ND
KGF	Incr in dermis	KGFR	Incr	IL-1α/β, TGF-α, Injury
IGF-1	ND	IGF-1R	Incr	ND
TGF-β$_1$	Normal	TGFβR1-3	ND	–

ND = Not done.

6.1.1 *Interleukin-1 (IL-1)*

IL-1 (and TNF-α) can be regarded as a "primary" cytokine because its release induces inflammation via pleiotropic effects such as the induction of adhesion molecules on endothelium and the production of a variety of secondary cytokines such as IL-6 and GM-CSF which act on inflammatory leukocytes.

KC contain large amounts of stored IL-1 which can be released following injury to the epidermis. IL-1 occurs in two forms, IL-1α and IL-1β which are the products of separate genes[1] but which have almost identical biological activities. They are produced as precursors, but while pro-IL-1α is biologically active, the IL-1β precursor only becomes active after proteolytic cleavage. In monocytes, this cleavage is catalysed by the IL-1β-converting enzyme (ICE). However, since KC do not possess this enzyme it was concluded that they were unable to process pro-IL-1β to the active form.[2]

The IL-1 receptor antagonist (IL-1ra) binds to the IL-1 receptor (IL-1R) without transducing a signal thus inhibiting responsiveness to IL-1.[3] IL-1ra occurs in two intracellular iso-forms (icIL-1ra I and II) and in a secreted isoform (sIL-1ra). The intracellular forms present in the cytosol of KC may antagonise intracellular IL-1α by binding to IL-1R present on the nuclear membrane.[4]

Two types of IL-1R have been characterised in humans, type I (IL-1RI) which transduces IL-1-mediated signals and type II (IL-1RII) which, with its short cytoplasmic domain, appears to act as a decoy target for IL-1.[5] Both types of IL-1R bind all IL-1 ligands. In addition, the extracellular portions of both types of IL-1R may be shed and act as IL-1 inhibitors.[6]

The evidence suggests that there is dysregulation of the IL-1 system in psoriasis. However, the findings reported by various groups have been inconsistent. The first indication that psoriatic lesions contained a biologically active IL-1-like compound came from a study of neutrophil chemoattractant material in aqueous extracts of lesional psoriatic scale.[7] Furthermore, staining of psoriatic skin with polyclonal antibodies revealed the presence of both forms, with a predominance of IL-1α which was mostly observed in the KC cytoplasm. In contrast, IL-1α distribution in normal epidermis was intercellular.[8] However in further studies, IL-1α was not detectable by immunofluorescence,[9] whilst IL-1β was absent from psoriatic blister fluid but overexpressed on the plasma membrane and in the intracellular compartment of psoriatic epidermal cells.[10] Similarly, IL-1ra has been reported to be decreased,[11] or conversely the ratio of IL-1ra to IL-1α protein signifi-cantly increased in lesional psoriatic compared to normal skin.[12]

Cooper *et al.* confirmed the presence of IL-1β in cytosolic extracts of psoriatic lesions and detected an increase in both the protein and its mRNA compared to that of normal skin.[9] However, in contrast to the earlier findings, this group reported a significant reduction in levels of immunoreactive IL-1α and of IL-1 activity in the same extracts (all IL-1 activity was attributable to IL-1α since IL-1β was shown to be non-functional).

The first evidence that psoriatic KC can produce bioactive IL-1β was provided by non-stimulated, short-term primary cultures (psoriatic epidermal cells *ex vivo*) which produced enhanced levels of biologically active IL-1α and IL-1β in a ratio of 3 : 1 whilst normal epidermal cells only released bioactive IL-1α.[13] The biological activity of Il-1β was confirmed in partially purified preparations of IL-1β from psoriatic scale in which an apparently total separation of IL-1β and IL-1ra had been achieved.[14] The mechanism of activation of IL-1β was thought to be similar to that present in non-inflamed plantar stratum corneum which does not involve ICE.[15]

In an effort to clarify the role of IL-1 in psoriasis, Debets *et al.* used an approach aimed at integrating different types of samples and techniques to determine the epidermal expression of all the currently known factors of the IL-1 system in psoriatic lesional skin.[16] They found by immunostaining that IL-1α was decreased to negligible levels in the psoriatic epidermis, whilst IL-1ra and IL-1RII were both significantly overexpressed in the suprabasal and basal compart-ments, respectively. Thus, an inverse correlation existed between the expression of IL-1α and of these two IL-1 antagonists which may be inherent to the accelerated terminal differentiation of the psoriatic

KC. Increased expression of IL-1β was also demonstrated using the more sensitive PCR technique, which was suggested to be related to the inflammatory response in psoriasis. Thus, in lesional psoriatic epidermis, there is a predominance of IL-1 antagonists which represents a negative feedback response to IL-1 agonists; the net result is a decrease in IL-1 responsiveness.

6.1.2 Interleukin-6 (IL-6)

IL-6 (formerly known as interferon β₂ or B cell stimulatory factor-2) plays a central role in the host response to injury and infection, and in haematopoiesis.[17] In common with IL-1, IL-6 exerts a multiplicity of effects on many types of target cells. These include stimulation of the production of acute-phase proteins by the liver, enhancement of the proliferation of B and T cell lines, induction of B cell differentiation and immunoglobulin production, and stimulation of cytotoxic T cells and NK cells via the induction of IL-2.

The expression of IL-6 protein is markedly increased in lesional psoriatic skin from patients with active disease, both in the epidermis and in inflammatory dermal cells compared to uninvolved skin from the same patients.[18] IL-6-specific immunostaining of cultured psoriatic and normal KC, and the detection of IL-6-specific mRNA in psoriatic epidermis by in situ hybridisation support the increased synthesis of IL-6 by proliferating KC in psoriatic lesions.[18]

Although one study failed to detect IL-6 by immunostaining and demonstrated only very low levels of IL-6 mRNA in KC from psoriatic lesions,[10] two other groups confirmed the increased production of IL-6 by psoriatic KC in active psoriasis.[19,20] No information is given regarding the activity or extent of disease of the patients in the negative study; it is possible that these patients had stable rather than active psoriasis which could explain the lack of increased IL-6 production.

In addition, circulating levels of IL-6 were also raised in patients with active psoriasis; this probably represents cytokine released from lesional skin.[18,20]

IL-6-specific receptors have been quantitated on normal KC.[21] It is therefore likely that IL-6 exerts both autocrine and paracrine effects within psoriatic lesions.

6.1.3 *Interleukin-7 (IL-7)*

IL-7 was originally identified as a growth factor for B cell progenitors,[22] but has subsequently been shown to exert a variety of effects including stimulation of the growth of T cell progenitors and mature peripheral T cells, activation of monocytes, induction of the production of cytokines (TNF-α, IL-4, GM-CSF, IFN-γ) and increase in CD25/IL-2 α-chain receptor expression on T lymphocytes.[23]

A recent study has shown that IL-7 levels are significantly increased in both biopsy and scale extracts obtained from lesional psoriatic compared to that of uninvolved psoriatic or normal skin.[24] In addition, serum levels were higher in these patients with active CP psoriasis than in the controls. In contrast, no differences were observed in the IL-7 levels in supernatants from unstimulated PBMC maintained in culture for 48 hours implying that the source of the cytokine may be psoriatic KC.[24] Indeed, normal human KC have been shown to express IL-7 mRNA and release IL-7 protein in biologically relevant amounts.[25]

IL-7 is upregulated in IFN-γ-stimulated KC which in turn (together with IL-2 and IL-12) stimulates IFN-γ production by T lymphocytes.[26] This is relevant to the increased IFN-γ concentrations in psoriatic lesional skin (see Sec. 3.2.3). Thus IL-7 is likely to play a significant role in the interaction between T cells and KC in psoriasis.

6.1.4 *Interleukin-8 (IL-8)*

IL-8 and melanoma growth-stimulatory activity (MGSA/gro) are heparin-binding 8 kD polypeptides which are potent neutrophil and/or T lymphocyte chemoattractants. They are members of a group of related cytokines which include IFN-γ-inducible protein (IP-10), platelet factor-4, β thromboglobulin and macrophage-derived inflammatory protein-2 (MIP-2) which share a cysteine-X-cysteine (C-X-C) motif near the amino terminus of the mature polypeptide and are thus designated as C-X-C proteins.[27] Three different gro genes have now been identified, α, β and γ which are 85–90% homologous at the protein level.[28] In contrast, another group of cytokines which have a cysteine-cysteine motif near the N terminus are designated the C–C proteins and are characterised by their inducibility by treatment with the "primary cytokines", for example, IL-1, TNF-α and IFN-γ.

Psoriatic scale was one of the first sources of the neutrophil-activating peptide, IL-8 and of other potent chemoattractants for neutrophils.[29] Interestingly, IL-8 immunoreactivity of psoriatic epidermis exhibited variable patterns of distribution which were related to disease activity and extent of inflammatory infiltration[30] or to the presence of TNF-α-positive dermal dendrocytes in the dermal papillae immediately below the IL-8-positive basal KC.[31] IL-8 mRNA, however, was confined to the very upper layers of epidermis and/ or parakeratotic stratum corneum in focal clusters.[32] Furthermore, KC from psoriatic skin exhibited a 10–20-fold increase in IL-8 production compared to normal KC.[33] In keeping with the ability of IL-8 to affect various functions of KC (see Sec. 6.2), the latter express IL-8 receptors (IL-8R) whose specific mRNA expression is increased 10 fold in lesional psoriatic epidermis.[34] (The possibility that this massive increase in expression of IL-8R was caused by neutrophil contamination was excluded.)

Northern blot analysis of RNA extracted from keratome biopsies of psoriatic skin revealed a significant correlation between levels of mRNA specific for gro and IL-8.[35] RT-PCR analysis showed that gro-α was predominant being approximately 6-fold more abundant than gro-β, and 25-fold more more abundant than gro-γ.[35] The significance of this differential gro expression is not known at present.

In addition, another member of this chemotactic and growth-promoting cytokine family, IP-10, is also more highly expressed in lesional psoriatic than in uninvolved psoriatic or normal epidermis.[36]

6.1.5 *Interleukin-10 (IL-10)*

IL-10 was originally identified as a cytokine synthesis inhibitor factor produced by activated T cell clones and immortalised B cells which acted upon TH_1 cells, probably by decreasing APC function through down-regulation of MHC Class II expression.[37] Subsequently, it was found that IL-10 could exert various effects including inhibition of macrophage-dependent proliferation of T lymphocytes, stimulation of B cells, and the ability to act as a chemoattractant for $CD8^+$ T cells and an inhibitor of IL-8-induced $CD4^+$ T cell migration.[38]

Human KC do not produce IL-10 under normal conditions[39] but can be induced to synthesize the cytokine by tape-stripping or by application of a recall antigen such as poison ivy antigen.[40] Although IL-10 was not detected by immunostaining in psoriatic epidermis,[40] IL-10 mRNA has been detected in psoriatic lesions by RT-PCR.[41] This may arise from macrophage-like cells in the dermis which, unlike psoriatic KC, stain positively for the cytokine.[40] Furthermore, functional receptors for IL-10 have recently been demonstrated on normal human KC;[42] the expression of such receptors is dramatically decreased in acute lesional but not uninvolved psoriatic epidermis as shown by *in vitro* and *in situ* binding, as well as RT-PCR studies.[42] These authors also demonstrated that IL-8, which is present in elevated concentrations in psoriatic lesions, is able to markedly reduce the IL-10R mRNA content in cultured epidermal cells, providing a possible explanation for the observations.

6.1.6 *Interleukin-12 (IL-12)*

IL-12 is a heterodimeric molecule composed of two covalently linked chains, p40 and p35, which have no biological activity alone (reviewed by Trinchieri).[43] The p35 chain of IL-12 is expressed by numerous, including non-lymphoid, cell types whilst the p40 IL-12 chain was thought to be restricted to the lymphoid cell system. IL-12 is a potent inducer of IFN-γ in T and NK cells, a growth factor for preactivated T and NK cells, and an enhancer of cytotoxic activity in both $CD8^+$

T cells and NK cells. APC-produced IL-12 plays a critical role in the generation of TH$_1$ cells and in the optimal differentiation of cytotoxic T cells.

In addition to phagocytic cells, B cells and other APC types, normal human KC also produce small amounts of IL-12. However, there has been conflicting reports as to whether mRNA specific for the p35[44], p40[45] or both[46] chains are constitutively expressed. *In situ*, the p35 chain mRNA was constitutively expressed and the p40 chain mRNA was only detected in epidermis treated with contact allergen.[44] In contrast, in cultured epidermal cells, p40 mRNA was amplified by RT-PCR but p35 mRNA was detectable only after phorbol-12,13-dibutyrate (PDBu) treatment.[45] Using a highly sensitive nested RT-PCR method, both IL-12 p35 and p40 transcripts were detected in normal KC cultures. In addition, low levels of the IL-12 p70 heterodimer were detected in culture supernatants by a sensitive ELISA.[46]

Both p35 and p40 IL-12 mRNA have been detected by RT-PCR in the epidermis of normal skin and psoriatic lesions, but the levels of p40 mRNA were considerably higher in the latter.[47] Furthermore, immunoreactivity for IL-12 p70 was markedly increased in psoriatic lesions and predominately expressed on mononuclear cells in the dermis.[47] These findings are compatible with the high levels of IFN-γ found in psoriatic lesions.

6.1.7 *Interleukin-15 (IL-15) and Interleukin-18 (IL-18)*

IL-15 is a cytokine with similar functions to that of IL-2, that is, it stimulates T cell proliferation and activates NK cells. However, unlike IL-2, IL-15 is not produced by T cells but by monocytes/macrophages, dermal fibroblasts and KC. Although not constitutively expressed by KC, IL-15 mRNA expression is induced by UVB treatment.[48]

IL-18 (IFN-γ-inducing factor) is another novel growth and differentiation factor for TH$_1$ cells with similar functions to that of IL-12. In common with IL-12, it is produced by macrophages, but also by contact allergen stimulated (murine) KC.[49]

Neither of these recently described cytokines have yet been studied in psoriatic lesions, but it would not be surprising if they are found to play a role in a disease in which the interaction between KC and T lymphocytes is central to the pathogenesis.

6.1.8 *Tumour Necrosis Factor-α (TNF-α)*

TNF-α is a multifunctional cytokine produced mainly by activated macrophages, T cells and mast cells, and also by KC after stimulation with endotoxin or UV light.[50] Its wide range of biological effects include endotoxic shock mediation, necrosis of transplanted tumours, cytotoxicity, growth modulation of normal cells and inflammatory, immunoregulatory and anti-viral responses.

Investigation of the presence of TNF-α in psoriatic lesions has produced conflicting results.[31,51] In the first study, intense and diffuse immunostaining for TNF-α was observed in lesional but not normal skin in dendrocytes (macrophages) in the papillary dermis, together with focal expression by KC and intraepidermal LCs.[31] In the second, staining for TNF-α was increased and distributed throughout the epidermis, but was strongest in basal KC and specifically localised to upper dermal blood vessels.[51] These differences in distribution of staining may be related to the specificity of the polyclonal anti-TNF-α antibodies used in each case. TNF-α immunoreactivity and bioactivity have also been shown to be consistently higher in lesional compared with uninvolved stratum corneum extracts.[52] This contrasted with two earlier studies in which lesional scale was found to be devoid of TNF-α immunoreactivity and/or biological activity.[53,54]

TNF-α exerts its biological effects via two immunologically distinct TNF-α receptors (TNFR) of approximately 55 kDa (TNF-R1) and 75 kDa (TNF-R2) which are independently regulated and have dissimilar cytoplasmic domains. In addition, TNF-R1 and TNF-R2 are differentially expressed on different cell types with, for example, preferential expression of TNF-R2 on activated T cells and of TNF-R1 on KC.[55]

In lesional psoriatic epidermis, TNF-R1 is distributed throughout the layers and in the parakeratotic stratum corneum and is predominately intracellular with perinuclear distribution.[51,56] This pattern is no different from that of normal skin except for an upregulation of expression of TNF-R1 in association with upper dermal blood vessels.[51] In contrast, TNF-R2 is not expressed by either normal or psoriatic epidermis.[51] Concentrations of soluble TNFRs are higher in lesional than uninvolved psoriatic stratum corneum extracts with a predominance of TNF-R1.[52] Elevated levels of soluble TNF-R1 were also detected in the plasma of psoriatic patients compared to those in normal controls which may help to regulate the effects of TNF-α in psoriasis.[52]

6.1.9 *Growth Factors*

6.1.9.1 *Transforming growth factor-α (TGF-α)/Epidermal growth factor (EGF)*

TGF-α is a polypeptide which is structurally related to EGF and binds to the EGF receptor (EGFR). TGF-α has a variety of effects including induction of tumour cell growth and oncogene expression, promotion of angiogenesis and induction of wound healing. TGF-α was initially regarded as an embryonic growth factor which is inappropriately expressed during neoplasia until it was discovered that primary cultures of normal, human KC synthesize TGF-α.[57] Furthermore, the addition of EGF or TGF to the cultures enhanced the levels of TGF-α mRNA expression demonstrating auto-induction.

Analysis of normal skin biopsies using *in situ* hybridisation (ISH) and immunohistochemistry confirmed the *in vivo* presence of both TGF-α mRNA and protein in the epidermis.[57] Strikingly, TGF-α in lesional psoriatic epidermis is markedly overexpressed compared to both uninvolved psoriatic and normal epidermis as shown by levels of specific mRNA and protein in epidermal extracts,[58] or by ISH (upper epidermal layers) and immunohistochemistry (upper and basal layers).[59] In addition, EGFR are also overexpressed in the hyperproliferative psoriatic epidermis as shown by ^{125}I-EGF binding to psoriatic skin.[60]

6.1.9.2 *Amphiregulin (AR)/Heparin-binding EGF-like growth factor (HB-EGF)*

AR and HB-EGF are heparin-binding polypeptide growth factors of the EGF family which are involved in the autocrine growth of cultured human KC via interaction with EGFRs.[61] Indeed, quantitatively AR may account for most of the autocrine growth capacity of cultured KC exceeding the contribution of TGF-α and HB-EGF. The expression of AR and HB-EGF is low to undetectable in normal epidermis but AR is upregulated in psoriasis and other epidermal hyperproliferative pathologies.[62] Interestingly, transgenic expression of the human AR gene in the basal KC of mice correlated with a psoriasis-like skin phenotype.[63] The majority (but it should be stressed, not all) of the clinical and histological features of psoriasis were reproduced, whereas transgenic epidermal overexpression of TGF-α induced only acanthosis and hyperkeratosis.[64] These findings suggest that overexpression of AR in the epidermis may contribute to the pathogenic process but is likely to be secondary to immune cell infiltration and activation *in situ* in patients with psoriasis.

6.1.9.3 *Keratinocyte growth factor (KGF)*

KGF is a fibroblast-derived member of the fibroblast growth factor (FGF) family (designated FGF-7) that represents another potent mitogen for epidermal KC. The KGF receptor (KGFR) is a transmembrane tyrosine kinase that is a splice variant of the FGFR-2 gene, and binds both KGF and acidic FGF with high affinity and basic FGF at low affinity. KGFR is expressed only by epithelial cells whereas FGFR-2 is present on a variety of different cell types. After wounding of skin, there is marked upregulation of KGF expression in fibroblasts below and at the edge of the wound.[65]

Similarly, both KGF and KGFR mRNA levels were shown to be elevated in the dermis and epidermis respectively, in psoriatic compared to normal skin.[66]

6.1.9.4 *Insulin-like growth factor-I (IGF-I) receptor*

IGF-I, previously termed somatomedin C, is a 7.5 kD polypeptide present in most tissues and in high concentrations in the plasma. It functions predominately as a mitogenic factor for various cell types via interaction with the IGF-IR which is composed of two subunits: α, a 125 kD protein that is extracellular and binds ligand, and β, a 95 kD transmembrane protein with extracellular and cytoplasmic domains. The IGF-IR, which is assembled into a heterodimer of both subunits ($\alpha_2\beta_2$), exhibits high affinity for IGF-I but also low and intermediate affinity for binding of insulin and IGF-II (members of the same family of structurally related hormones), respectively. In KC, IGF-I regulates proliferation via synergistic interactions with EGF- or FGF-like factors. However, the IGF-IR distribution is different from that of the EGFR being restricted to the basal KC of normal skin. In psoriasis, in common with EGFR, there is an overexpression of the IGF-IR and, furthermore, the IGF-IR pathway is activated as suggested by the measurement of IGF-I kinase activity.[67] Activation of increased IGF-IR in lesional psoriatic skin by IGF released from leaky capillaries or secreted by dermal fibroblasts might increase EGFR expression via IGF-I-mediated transmodulation of the EGFR.[68]

6.1.9.5 *Transforming growth factor-β (TGF-β)*

TGF-β, a homodimer, is a member of a complex family of structurally related growth and differentiation factors. Three subtypes, TGF-β_1, TGF-β_2 and TGF-β_3 have been described which are present in various combinations in most nucleated cell types. The expressed proteins are biologically inactive and must be cleaved to form active dimers. The various forms of TGF-β bind to a set of three structurally and functionally distinct cell surface receptors present on most cell types — high affinity types I and II, and low affinity type III. The type I and type II receptors are thought to associate to mediate signal transduction events.

Although TGF-β stimulates proliferation of some fibroblast cell types in culture, it has a growth inhibitory effect on epithelial cells. In addition, TGF-β modulates lymphocyte function by suppressing IL-2 activity and inhibiting lymphocyte proliferation.

In contrast to overexpression of TGF-α, TGF-β_1 mRNA levels were not found to be significantly different in normal, uninvolved or lesional psoriatic epidermis.[58] A study of the levels of TGF-βR has not, as far as is known, been carried out on psoriatic skin.

6.1.10 *Monocyte Chemotactic Protein-1 (MCP-1)/Monocyte Chemoattractant and Activating Factor (MCAF)*

In contrast to the presence of neutrophils and T lymphocytes in the epidermis of psoriatic lesions, macrophages appear to be almost exclusively restricted to the papillary dermis and arranged along the rete ridges in close proximity to proliferating KC. In correlation with this distribution, ISH revealed strong signals for mRNA specific for the potent monocyte chemoattractant MCP-1 over the proliferating basal KC of the tips of the rete ridges and, to a lesser extent, in cells in the dermal papillae.[69] In contrast, a lower expression for MCP-1 mRNA was detected in uninvolved psoriatic or normal skin.[69]

6.2 Response to Cytokines

6.2.1 *Increased Proliferation*

Normal human KC proliferation can be stimulated *in vitro* by a variety of cytokines including IL-6, IL-8, TGF-α (EGF) and possibly IL-1 and GM-CSF.[18,70–73] However, it appears that the culture conditions in which the cells are grown plays an important part in the type and degree of response. Thus, IL-6 was stimulatory for normal KC

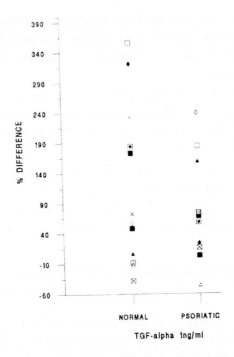

Fig. 6.1. Proliferation of 12 normal and 10 psoriatic KC cultures stimulated with TGF-α for four days. Data expressed as % difference in cpm (tritiated thymidine incorporation) with and without cytokine. (Source: Olaniran A.K. *et al.*, A comparison of the stimulatory effects of cytokines on normal and psoriatic keratinocytes *in vitro*, *Arch.Dermatol.Res.* **287** (1995), 231–236, Fig. 2, with permission from Springer-Verlag GmbH & Co., Heidelberg, Germany.)

proliferation when cultured in a serum-free system,[18] but no cytokine-induced growth was seen in a serum supplemented system.[74]

A comparison of the stimulatory effects of various cytokines on normal and psoriatic KC proliferation *in vitro*, using a serum-free culture system, revealed that psoriatic KC were equally responsive to TGF-α (Fig. 6.1) and IL-8, but less susceptible to IL-6 than normal KC.[75] However, only two psoriatic KC cultures did not respond to IL-6 and they showed a marked rate of proliferation in basal medium alone suggesting that they were already maximally stimulated. Thus, further studies are required to establish whether psoriatic KC are truly less susceptible to the proliferative effects of IL-6. Both normal and psoriatic KC were shown to be generally unresponsive to the effects of GM-CSF.[75] This contrasts with the findings of an earlier study.[73]

6.2.2 Decreased Proliferation

Reversible inhibition of normal human KC proliferation can be induced by the cytokines TNF-α, TGF-β, IFN-γ and IL-10.[42,76–78] Psoriatic KC show a normal response to the inhibitory effects of TNF-α and TGF-β (Fig. 6.2).[56] Response to IL-10 by psoriatic KC

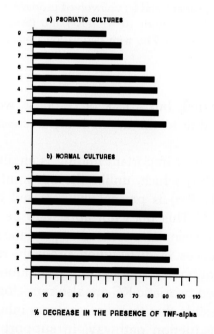

a) PSORIATIC CULTURES

b) NORMAL CULTURES

0 10 20 30 40 50 60 70 80 90 100 110

% DECREASE IN THE PRESENCE OF TNF-alpha

Fig. 6.2. Percentage decrease in thymidine incorporation of (a) 9 psoriatic and (b) 10 normal KC cultures in the presence versus absence of 20 ng/ml TNF-α after 3–4 days incubation. (Source: Malkani A.K. *et al. Exp.Dermatol.* **2** (1993), 224–230, with permission from Munksgaard, Copenhagen, Denmark.)

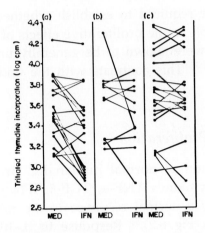

Fig. 6.3. IFN-γ-induced inhibition of tritiated thymidine incorporation (log cpm) in (a) normal, (b) lesional psoriatic and (c) uninvolved psoriatic epidermal cell cultures after seven days incubation with 10^2 U IFN-γ/ml. (Source: Baker B.S. *et al.*, *Scand.J.Immunol.* **28** (1988), 735–740, with permission from Blackwell Science Ltd, Oxford, UK.)

has not been reported, but a lack of response would be expected in acute psoriasis due to the dramatically decreased expression of IL-10R.[42]

The potentially most important finding is an altered response by psoriatic KC to IFN-γ which, unlike the other inhibitory cytokines (except perhaps TNF-α) is present in increased quantities in skin lesions (Fig. 6.3).[79,80] This does not appear to be due to a lack of IFN-γR as they have been demonstrated on psoriatic KC by two groups albeit with differences in distribution probably resulting from the use of different antibodies and staining techniques.[81,82]

Since uninvolved psoriatic KC are also refractory to inhibition by IFN-γ,[79,80] it is possible that this represents an inherent defect in the IFN-γ signal transduction pathway. In support of these *in vitro* findings, injection of IFN-γ into psoriatic patients either intralesionally or systemically, failed to inhibit DNA synthesis in psoriatic epidermis as measured by autoradiography.[83]

6.2.3 *Surface Molecule Expression*

The interaction between T lymphocytes and KC in psoriatic epidermis involves predominately lymphocyte function-associated antigen-1 (LFA-1) and its ligand the cell surface glycoprotein, intercellular adhesion molecule-1 (ICAM-1; CD54), respectively. ICAM-1 is not normally expressed by KC but can be upregulated by IFN-γ and TNF-α which act in synergy.[84,85] In psoriasis, KC ICAM-1 expression is focal and localised at the tips of the papillary dermis containing large numbers of activated (HLA-DR+) T cells, which correlates well with the presence of intraepidermal LFA-1+ T cells.[85]

In addition to ICAM-1, IFN-γ induces MHC Class II (predominately HLA-DR and HLA-DQ), a Class II-like molecule HLA-DM, and invariant chain expression by KC which normally lack or express low levels of these molecules.[86,87] All of these molecules are required for the generation of functional Class II/peptide complexes for presentation to T cells. In psoriatic lesions, however, HLA-DR expression has been observed only infrequently[31,88] and was only detected in highly inflamed portions of psoriatic lesions such as early pin-point lesions or margins of active plaque lesions.[89] The induction of HLA-DR expression by IFN-γ on psoriatic KC *in vitro* has been reported to be the same[80] or decreased[79] compared to that of uninvolved psoriatic or normal KC. However, intralesional injection of IFN-γ induced the expression of HLA-DR antigen in both uninvolved and involved psoriatic epidermis *in vivo*.[83] In addition, IL-8 can also induce HLA-DR expression by KC whilst IL-10 inhibits the induction of HLA-DR by IFN-γ.[42]

Recently, it has been demonstrated that CD40, a member of the TNF-α superfamily, is in addition to lymphoid cells functionally expressed by normal human KC.[90,91] The CD40/gp39 pathway is known to be an important feature of B/T cell collaboration leading to activation, proliferation or differentiation of B cells.

In KC, CD40 is markedly upregulated following stimulation with IFN-γ, but not with TNF-α or IL-1β. Activation of KC cell surface CD40 by monoclonal anti-CD40 or ligation with soluble gp39, the

CD40 ligand (CD40L), led to an increase in secretion of IL-6, IL-8 and TNF-α by the activated KC and upregulation of ICAM-1 and Bcl-x, an inhibitor of apoptosis (programmed cell death).[90-92] Furthermore, ligation of KC CD40 by CD40L-transfected L cells or by soluble CD40L led to inhibition of KC proliferation which correlated with differentiation of the cells.[92]

In psoriasis, KC display a markedly enhanced expression of CD40 which colocalises with the expression of ICAM-1, Bcl-x and an influx of CD3+ T cells.[91]

Another molecule which is expressed on psoriatic KC, but is restricted to melanocytes in normal skin, is CDw60[93] which is present on approximately 25% of peripheral blood T cells (and 75% of T cells in psoriatic lesions), and is involved in T cell activation. The UM4D4 antibody which detects CDw60 has been shown to bind to the o-acetylated form of ganglioside G_{D3}, especially the 9-0-acetylated form.[94] Gangliosides are sialylated glycosphingolipids located in the plasma membrane which are thought to play a role in the control of cell proliferation and differentiation, as well as in cell surface recognition.

6.2.4 *Cytokine Production*

The interaction of various cytokines with their specific receptors present on KC leads to induction of their own production (e.g. TNF-α) and/or to the production of other cytokines (e.g. the induction of IL-8 by TNF-α). Alternatively, one cytokine may lead to down-regulation of the receptors for a different cytokine such as Il-8 and IL-10R., respectively. It is also clear that cytokines do not act in isolation, a good example of which is the synergy demonstrated between the effects induced by IFN-γ and TNF-α. The details of how one cytokine affects the function of another within the psoriatic process have not been examined as yet. However, the variety of cytokines detected in skin lesions suggest that it is likely to be very complex.

6.3 Antigen/Superantigen Presentation

As KC are induced to express MHC Class II antigens and accessory proteins in response to IFN-γ, there is a possibility that these cells can act as APC to T cells. Recognition of antigen presented by specialised APC such as macrophages or dendritic cells leads to T cell activation. In contrast, antigen presentation by cells which lack accessory function can lead to a state of specific non-responsiveness, characterised by a failure of T cells to produce IL-2.

When IFN-γ-induced DR4 expressing KC were used to present specific peptide to a HLA-DR1/4-restricted influenza haemagglutinin-specific T cell clone, the T cells became tolerised and were unable to proliferate.[95] The induction of T cell tolerance was both antigen-specific and HLA-DR-restricted. These findings suggested that HLA-DR⁺ KC did not provide the accessory or second signals required for T cell activation. However, subsequently, using a sensitive assay system employing intact layers of basal KC as APC, Mutis *et al.*[96] was able to demonstrate that HLA-DR⁺ KC could present *M.leprae* antigens to well-defined cytotoxic as well as proliferative CD4⁺ TH₁-like cell clones and induce them to secrete IFN-γ in an antigen-specific and HLA Class II-restricted manner. Thus, in this system, HLA Class II-positive KC were functioning as proper APC and, furthermore, appeared to be able to process antigen into peptides.

About this time, it was reported that activated KC express BB-1, a ligand for CD28 expressed by T cells.[97] BB-1 is one of a family of B7 molecules expressed by professional APC (macrophages, B cells, dendritic cells) which, on binding to CD28, delivers a co-stimulatory signal required for optimal activation of T cells via the TCR/CD3 complex. Furthermore, it was shown that IFN-γ-treated KC can, under appropriate conditions, provide costimulation for superantigen-activated T cells inducing their proliferation in the absence of other APCs.[98] However, this costimulation did not seem to be dependent upon activation of the CD28 pathway, since it was not blocked by antibodies directed at the CD28 ligand present on KC, BB-1. On the contrary, antibodies against LFA-1α or β, or against ICAM-1 significantly inhibited the response. In addition, when KC were used as APC, a specific defect in T cell IFN-γ production in response to the superantigen SEB was observed.[99] In contrast, IL-2 and IL-4 were produced at levels comparable with those seen when professional APCs which express B7.1 (CD80) or B7.2 (CD86) were used. The specific ability of KC to induce a TH$_2$ response was closely linked with an absence of IL-12 production, and addition of rIL-12 restored IFN-γ levels to those found in cultures containing professional APCs.[99]

The conflicting findings from the various studies probably arose from differences in culture conditions including the use of adherent versus supensions of KC, different numbers and ratios of T cells to KC, nature of antigen etc. However, it seems that if the conditions are optimal, HLA-DR⁺ KC do appear able to present antigen to T cells and induce their activation. Whether these criteria are met *in situ* within the psoriatic epidermis remains to be elucidated. Moreover, the question arises as to why it should be necessary for KC to act as APC in this situation when professional APC are present in abundance.

6.4 Integrins

The integrins are a family of heterodimeric membrane glycoproteins expressed on the cell surface and linked to the cytoskeleton which mediate cell-cell and cell-extracellular matrix adhesion, and transmit signals both into and out from cells.[100] Each integrin consists of two non-covalently associated subunits, α and β. At least 14 different α and 8 β subunits have been identified; several α chains can associate with a single β chain and, to a lesser extent, the reverse is also true (Table 6.2).

In human epidermis and stratified KC cultures, integrin expression is largely confined to the basal layer where they mediate cell adhesion and migration, and regulate stratification and the initiation of terminal differentiation.

Table 6.2   Integrin subunit associations

β Subunit	α Subunit
β_1	$\alpha_1-\alpha_7$
β_2	$\alpha_L, \alpha_M, \alpha_X$
β_3	α_V, α_{IIb}
β_4	α_6
β_5	α_V
β_6	α_V
β_7	α_4, α_E
β_8	α_V

Table 6.3   Integrin heterodimers expressed by normal keratinocytes and their ligands

Integrin Heterodimer	Ligand	Location
$\alpha_1\beta_1$ (weakly expressed)	Unknown	Basal KC
$\alpha_2\beta_1$	Collagen	Lateral surface of basal, & suprabasal KC
$\alpha_3\beta_1$	Laminin	Lateral surface of basal, & suprabasal KC
$\alpha_5\beta_1$ (weakly expressed)	Fibronectin	Basal KC plasma membrane
$\alpha_v\beta_5$	Vitronectin	Basal KC
$\alpha_6\beta_4$	Unknown	Basal aspect of basal KC, in Hemidesmosomes

Furthermore, integrin heterodimers are located to discrete KC membrane domains (Table 6.3). Thus, $\alpha_2\beta_1$ and $\alpha_3\beta_1$ integrins are concentrated in the lateral surface of basal and immediate by suprabasal KC, suggesting their role in cell-cell adhesion of epithelial cells. In contrast, $\alpha_6\beta_4$ integrin is strictly located to the basal aspect of the basal KC and is found in hemidesmosomes, suggesting a role as a basal lamina receptor.[101] This polarised distribution is markedly altered in KC from psoriatic skin, and during wound healing at the time of wound closure when the epidermis is still hyperproliferative, where integrin expression on suprabasal cells is observed.[102,103] In addition, the role of such integrins in mediating KC adhesion *in vitro* is modified. The integrin-cytoskeleton relationship was also found to be altered in psoriatic KC and, in contrast to normal KC, showed increased fibronectin receptor ($\alpha_5\beta_1$) staining *in vivo*.[102]

These alterations of expression, distribution and function of integrins were also observed in KC from uninvolved psoriatic skin.[102] Furthermore, fibronectin significantly increased cell cycle entry, and potentiated the expansion of uninvolved psoriatic KC, relative to normal KC, in response to a mixture of T cell cytokines.[104] These findings suggest that increased expression of the fibronectin receptor contributes to the hyperproliferation of KC in response to cytokines produced by intralesional T cells.

Various cytokines have been investigated as possible stimuli for suprabasal integrin expression but neither TGF-β, IFN-γ or TNF-α were able to induce such expression.[105] It is likely therefore that suprabasal integrin expression probably reflects the proliferation/ differentiation status of the epidermis which even in uninvolved psoriatic skin is altered compared to skin from non-psoriatic individuals.

When functional human integrin subunit β_1, alone or in combination with α_2 or α_5, was expressed in the suprabasal epidermal layers of transgenic mice, features of psoriasis, that is, epidermal hyperproliferation, perturbed KC differentiation and skin inflammation were observed.[106] The authors concluded that these findings strongly support the view that psoriasis is primarily a disorder of KC rather than of the immune system. However, it is more likely that both components are necessary as suggested by the synergistic effects of fibronectin and T cell cytokines.[104]

6.5 Apoptosis

Apoptosis (or programmed cell death) is an active process of cell deletion which can be differentiated from necrosis by characteristic features such as chromatin condensation, DNA fragmentation and blebbing of the plasma membrane. In addition, to embryogenesis, tissue atrophy and tumour regression, there is now convincing evidence that apoptosis occurs in normal skin contributing to epidermal homeostasis by removing excess cells and maintaining normal cell numbers. KC apoptosis has also been postulated to be involved in hair bulb cycling, response to sunburn, and prevention of neoplasia.

Apoptosis can be triggered by various factors including growth factor deprivation, detachment from extracellular matrix, UVB irradiation, stimulation with 1,25-dihydroxyvitamin D_3, TGF-β_1 or calcium, or by oligomerization of Fas (CD95) by the Fas ligand (FasL, CD95L) or anti-Fas.[107,108]

Fas antigen is a transmembrane molecule which belongs to the nerve growth factor/TNFR superfamily. Its corresponding ligand is a type II transmembrane protein that belongs to the TNF-α family which includes other cell surface molecules that promote (p55 TNF-αR) or prevent (CD40) apoptosis. FasL is found on activated T cells, but can also be induced on KC by UVB irradiation.[109] Although Fas antigen is expressed at low levels or not at all in normal, human epidermis, it is markedly upregulated on human KC in a number of inflammatory and infectious skin diseases, including psoriasis, and in response to culture with IFN-γ (Table 6.4).[108,110] In addition, the long form of Bcl-x (Bcl-x_L), but not Bcl-2, which both prevent apoptosis in lymphocytes, is also upregulated in psoriasis,[110] whilst the expression of potent inducers of cell death such as Bax and Bak have not been studied as yet.

In contrast to normal epidermis where occasional nuclei were positive, KC throughout all layers of lesional psoriatic epidermis were abundantly positive by the TdT-mediated dUTP-biotin nick end labelling (TUNEL) assay.[110] This assay is a highly sensitive

Table 6.4   Expression of pro- and anti-apoptotic proteins in normal and psoriatic epidermis

Proteins	Normal KC	Psoriatic KC	Upregulated By
Pro-apoptotic Fas	Minimal/absent	Upregulated	IFN-γ, TPA (tumor promotor)
FasL	Minimal/absent	Minimal/absent	UVB, TPA, IFN-γ, TNF-α
Anti-apoptotic Bcl-2	Minimal/absent	Minimal/absent	IL-10
Bcl-x_L	Minimal	Upregulated	IFN-γ, TPA
CD40	Basal	Upregulated	IFN-γ, TPA

immunostaining procedure designed to detect single strand 3'-OH DNA ends produced by DNA fragmentation which is used to detect cells under-going apoptosis. However, it was demonstrated subsequently that numerous TUNEL-positive KC in psoriatic plaques were also positive for proliferating cell nuclear antigen and Ki-67 antigen and possessed a DNA content profile indicative of proliferating and not dying cells.[111] In addition, freshly isolated psoriatic KC lacked double-stranded DNA fragmentation, a characteristic of apoptosis and, also exhibited a prolonged capacity to resist induction of apoptosis compared with normal KC.[111]

Thus, it appears that psoriatic KC are able to resist apoptosis, which is consistent with the accumulation of KC in psoriatic epidermis. However, the mechanisms involved are not clear. The increase in Bcl-x_L expression in psoriatic lesions may be sufficient to block cell death, but this molecule may not necessarily be anti-apoptotic in all situations. It has recently been reported that caspases, a family of cysteine proteases implicated in the biochemical and morphological changes that occur during apoptosis can convert Bcl-2 and Bcl-x_L into pro-apoptotic molecules.[112] Thus a detailed study of the apoptosis pathway in psoriatic KC is necessary.

References

1. March C.J. *et al. Nature (London)* **315** (1985), 641–647.
2. Mizutani H., Black R., Kupper T.S. *J.Clin.Invest.* **87** (1991), 1066–1071.
3. Eisenberg S.P. *Nature (London)* **343** (1990), 341–346.
4. Curtis B.M., Widmer M.B., De Roos P., Qwarnstrom E.E. *J.Immunol.* **144** (1990), 1295–1303.
5. Colotta F. *Science* **261** (1993), 472–475.
6. Symons J.A., Eastgate J.A., Duff G.W. *J.Exp.Med.* **174** (1991), 1251–1254.
7. Camp R.D.R. *J.Immunol.* **137** (1986), 3469–3474.
8. Romero L.I., Ikejima T., Pincus S.H. *J.Invest.Dermatol.* **93** (1989), 518–522.
9. Cooper K.D. *et al. J.Immunol.* **144** (1990), 4593–4603.
10. Prens E.P. *et al. J.Invest.Dermatol.* **95** (1990), 121S–124S.
11. Kristensen M. *et al. Br.J.Dermatol.* **127** (1992), 305–311.
12. Hammerberg C. *et al. J.Clin.Invest.* **90** (1992), 571–583.
13. Debets R. *et al. Eur.J.Immunol.* **25** (1995), 1624–1630.
14. Nylander Lundquist E. and Egelrud T. *Eur.J.Immunol.* **27** (1997), 2165–2171.
15. Nylander Lundquist E., Back O., Egelrud T. *J.Immunol.* **157** (1996), 1699–1704.
16. Debets R. *et al. J.Immunol.* **158** (1997), 2955–2963.
17. Barton B.E. *Med.Res.Rev.* **16** (1996), 87–109.
18. Grossman R.M. *et al. Proc.Natl.Acad.Sci. (USA)* **86** (1989), 6367–6371.
19. Oxholm A., Oxholm P., Staberg B., Bendtzen K. *Acta Derm.Venereol (Stockh)* **69** (1989), 195–199.
20. Neuner P. *et al. J.Invest.Dermatol.* **97** (1991), 27–33.
21. Krueger J.G., Krane J.F., Carter D.M., Gottlieb A.B. *J.Invest.Dermatol.* **94** (1990), 135S–140S.
22. Namen A.E. *et al. Nature (London)* **333** (1988), 571–573.
23. Costello R., Imbert J., Olive D. *Eur.Cytokine Network* **4** (1993), 253–262.
24. Bonifati C. *et al. Clin.Immunol.Immunopathol.* **83** (1997), 41–44.
25. Heufler C. *J.Exp.Med.* **178** (1993), 1109–1114.
26. Borger P., Kauffman H.F., Postma D.S., Vellenga E. *J.Immunol.* **156** (1996), 1333–1338.
27. Sager R. In *Molecular and Cellular Biology of Cytokines*, Oppenheim J.J. *et al.* (eds), Wiley-Liss, New York (1990), 327–332.

28. Haskill S. *et al. Proc.Natl.Acad.Sci. (USA)* **87** (1990), 7732–7736.
29. Schroder J.M. and Christophers E. *J.Invest.Dermatol.* **87** (1986), 53–58.
30. Sticherling M., Bornscheuer E., Schroder J.M., Christophers E. *J.Invest.Dermatol.* **96** (1991), 26–30.
31. Nickoloff B.J. *et al. Am.J.Pathol.* **138** (1991), 129–140.
32. Gillitzer R. *et al. J.Invest.Dermatol.* **97** (1991), 73–79.
33. Nickoloff B.J. *et al. Am.J.Pathol.* **144** (1994), 820–828.
34. Schulz B.S. *et al. J.Immunol.* **151** (1993), 4399–4406.
35. Kojima T. *et al. J.Invest.Dermatol.* **101** (1993), 767–772.
36. Gottlieb A.B., Luster A.D., Posnett D.N., Carter D.M. *J.Exp.Med.* **168** (1988), 941–948.
37. Fiorentino D.F. *et al. J.Immunol.* **146** (1991), 3444–3451.
38. Jinquan T. *et al. J.Immunol.* **151** (1993), 4545–4551.
39. Teunissen M.B.M. *Clin.Exp.Immunol.* **107** (1997), 213–223.
40. Nickoloff B.J. *et al. Clin.Immunol.Immunopathol.* **73** (1994), 63–68.
41. Olaniran A. *et al. Arch.Dermatol.Res.* **288** (1996), 421–425.
42. Michel G. *et al. J.Immunol.* **159** (1997), 6291–6297.
43. Trincheiri G. *Ann.Rev.Immunol.* **13** (1995), 251–276.
44. Muller G. *et al. J.Clin.Invest.* **94** (1994), 1799–1805.
45. Aragane Y. *et al. J.Immunol.* **153** (1994), 5366–5372.
46. Yawalkar N., Limat A., Brand C.U., Braathen L.R. *J.Invest.Dermatol.* **106** (1996), 80–83.
47. Yawalkar N. *et al. J.Invest.Dermatol.* **110** (1998), 665 (Abstract).
48. Mohamadzadeh M. *et al. J.Immunol.* **155** (1995), 4492–4496.
49. Stoll S. *et al. J.Immunol.* **159** (1997), 298–302.
50. Kock A. *et al. J.Exp.Med.* **172** (1990), 1609–1614.
51. Kristensen M. *et al. Clin.Exp.Immunol.* **94** (1993), 354–362.
52. Ettehadi P. *et al. Clin.Exp.Med.* **96** (1994), 146–151.
53. Takematsu H., Ohta H., Tagami H. *Arch.Dermatol.Res.* **281** (1989), 389–400.
54. Gearing A.J.H. *et al. Cytokine* **2** (1990), 68–75.
55. Trefzer U. *et al. J.Invest.Dermatol.* **97** (1991), 911–916.
56. Malkani A.K. *et al. Exp.Dermatol.* **2** (1993), 224–230.
57. Coffey R.J. *et al. Nature (London)* **328** (1987), 817–820.
58. Elder J.T. *et al. Science* **243** (1989), 811–814.
59. Turbitt M.L., Akhurst R.J., White S.I., Mackie R.M. *J.Invest.Dermatol.* **95** (1990), 229–232.

60. Nanney L.B., Stoscheck C.M., Magid M., King L.E. *J.Invest.Dermatol.* **86** (1986), 260–265.
61. Piepkorn M., Lo C., Plowman G. *J.Cell Physiol.* **159** (1994), 114–120.
62. Piepkorn M. *Am.J.Dermatopathol.* **18** (1996), 165–171.
63. Cook P.W. *et al. J.Clin.Invest.* **100** (1997), 2286–2294.
64. Dominey A.M. *et al. Cell Growth Diff.* **4** (1993), 1071–1082.
65. Marchese C. *et al. J.Exp.Med.* **182** (1995), 1369–1376.
66. Finch P.W., Murphy F., Cardinale I., Krueger J.G. *Am.J.Pathol.* **151** (1997), 1619–1628.
67. Krane J.F., Gottlieb A.B., Carter D.M., Krueger J.G. *J.Exp.Med.* **175** (1992), 1081–1090.
68. Krane J.F., Murphy D.P., Carter D.M., Krueger J.G. *J.Invest.Dermatol.* **96** (1991), 419–424.
69. Gillitzer R. *et al. J.Invest.Dermatol.* **101** (1993), 127–131.
70. Tuschil A., Lam C., Haslberger A., Lindley I. *J.Invest.Dermatol.* **99** (1992), 294–298.
71. Barrandon Y. and Green H. *Cell* **50** (1987), 1131–1137.
72. Ristow H.J. *Proc.Natl.Acad.Sci (USA)* **84** (1987), 1940–1944.
73. Hancock G.E., Kaplan G., Cohn Z.A. *J.Exp.Med.* **168** (1988), 1395–1402.
74. Partridge M., Chantry D., Turner M., Feldmann M. *J.Invest.Dermatol.* **96** (1991), 771–776.
75. Olaniran A.K. *et al. Arch.Dermatol.Res.* **287** (1995), 231–236.
76. Detmar M. and Orfanos C.E. *Arch.Dermatol.Res.* **282** (1990), 238–245.
77. Shipley G.D. *et al. Cancer Res.* **46** (1986), 2068–2071.
78. Nickoloff B.J., Basham T.Y., Merigan T.C., Morhenn V.B. *Lab.Invest.* **51** (1984), 697–701.
79. Baker B.S., Powles A.V., Valdimarsson H., Fry L. *Scand.J.Immunol.* **28** (1988), 735–740.
80. Nickoloff B.J. *et al. Br.J.Dermatol.* **121** (1989), 161–174.
81. Scheynius A. *et al. J.Invest.Dermatol.* **98** (1992), 255–258.
82. Van den Oord J.J., DeLey M., De Wolf-Peeters C. *Path.Res.Pract.* **191** (1995), 530–534.
83. Schulze H.-J. and Mahrle G. *Arch.Dermatol.Res.* **278** (1986), 416–418.
84. Dustin M.L., Singer K.H., Tuck D.T., Springer T.A. *J.Exp.Med.* **167** (1988), 1323–1340.
85. Griffiths C.E.M., Voorhees J.J., Nickoloff B.J. *J.Am.Acad.Dermatol.* **20** (1989), 617–629.

86. Basham T.Y., Nickoloff B.J., Merigan T.C., Morhenn V.B. *J.Invest.Dermatol.* **83** (1984), 88–90.
87. Albanesi C., Cavani A., Girolomoni G. *J.Invest.Dermatol.* **110** (1998), 138–142.
88. Aubock J., Romani N., Grubauer G., Fritsch P. *Br.J.Dermatol.* **114** (1986), 465–472.
89. Terui T. *et al. Br.J.Dermatol.* **116** (1987), 87–93.
90. Gaspari A.A. *et al. Eur.J.Immunol.* **26** (1996), 1371–1377.
91. Denfeld R.W. *et al. Eur.J.Immunol.* **26** (1996), 2329–2334.
92. Peguet-Navarro J. *et al. J.Immunol.* **158** (1997), 144–152.
93. Skov L. *et al. Am.J.Pathol.* **150** (1997), 675–683.
94. Kniep B. *et al. Biochem.Biophys.Res.Commun.* **187** (1992), 1343–1349.
95. Bal V. *et al. Eur.J.Immunol.* **20** (1990), 1893–1897.
96. Mutis T., De Bueger M., Bakker A., Ottenholff T.H.M. *Scand.J.Immunol.* **37** (1993), 43–51.
97. Nickoloff B.J. *et al. Am.J.Pathol.* **142** (1993), 1029–1040.
98. Nickoloff B.J. *et al.J.Immunol.* **150** (1993), 2148–2159.
99. Goodman R.E. *et al. J.Immunol.* **152** (1994), 5189–5198.
100. Hynes R.O. *Cell* **48** (1987), 549–554.
101. Marchisio P.C. *et al. J.Cell Biol.* **112** (1991), 761–773.
102. Pellegrini G. *et al. J.Clin.Invest.* **89** (1992), 1783–1795.
103. Hertle M., Kubler M.-D., Leigh I.M., Watt F.M. *J.Clin.Invest.* **89** (1992), 1892–1901.
104. Bata-Csorgo Z. *et al. J.Clin.Invest.* **101** (1998), 1509–1518.
105. Hertle M.D. *et al. J.Invest.Dermatol.* **104** (1995), 260–265.
106. Carroll J.M., Romero M.R., Watt F.M. *Cell* **83** (1995), 957–968.
107. Benassi L. *et al. J.Invest.Dermatol.* **109** (1997), 276–282.
108. Sayami K., Yonehara S., Watanabe Y., Miki Y. *J.Invest.Dermatol.* **103** (1994), 330–334.
109. Gutierrez-Steil C. *et al. J.Clin.Invest.* **101** (1998), 33–39.
110. Wrone-Smith T. *et al. Am.J.Pathol.* **146** (1995), 1079–1088.
111. Wrone-Smith T. *et al. Am.J.Pathol.* **151** (1997), 1321–1329.
112. Cheng E.H.-Y. *et al. Science* **278** (1997), 1966–1968.

CHAPTER 7

Current and Future Immunological Approaches to Treatment of Psoriasis

Current immunosuppressive treatments for psoriasis provide only temporary respite as skin lesions appear again shortly after treatment is stopped. In addition, their effects are non-specific and thus their dampening down of the immune system inevitably incurs side-effects which can vary from mild effects such as headaches and nausea to renal- or nephro-toxicity and increased risk of skin cancer. In contrast, the novel pharmacologic and biological agents of the future have to be firstly, specifically directed against the disease-inducing pathogenic MHC/antigen/T cell complex to avoid global effects, and secondly, be capable of inducing a long-lasting tolerance to the triggering antigen(s).

The mechanisms of action of current treatments will be discussed. This will be followed by a description of the various novel approaches now being applied to the treatment of various autoimmune diseases. Some of these approaches are currently being tested in psoriasis; others are likely to be suitable candidates for clinical trials when more information concerning the antigen specificity of the pathogenic T cells in psoriatic skin lesions becomes known.

7.1 Current Treatments

Current treatments for psoriasis include UV light (UVB and PUVA), cyclosporin A (CyA) and FK506, vitamin D and A analogues, corticosteroids, methotrexate and dithranol which are used singly and in various combinations to reduce individual doses and, therefore, side-effects. These therapies mostly act as immunosuppressants, but may also have effects on KC and/or other cell types in the skin. Table 7.1 shows the mechanism of action of these current treatments on T cells and KC. It should be noted that APC are also affected by most of these treatment modalities.

7.1.1 *PUVA and UVB*

Treatment of psoriasis with either PUVA or UVB results in clinical resolution preceded or accompanied by a reduction in CD4[+] and CD8[+] T cell numbers in the epidermis.[1,2] Repeated exposure of psoriatic skin lesions to PUVA, but not UVB, results in a marked depletion of epidermal LC numbers.[3] Furthermore, some LCs which remain after PUVA treatment have an altered morphology with a loss of HLA-DR antigen and a reduced ability to stimulate a mixed lymphocyte reaction *in vitro*.[4] These reductions in immune cell numbers are accompanied by decreases in specific mRNA and/or protein specific for cytokines such as IL-2, IL-6, IL-8, IFN-γ, TNF-α and TGF-α.[5-7]

Recently it has been demonstrated that the mechanism of action underlying the effectiveness of UVB in psoriasis is likely to be the induction of apoptosis in epidermal T cells.[2] KC, on the other hand, were not induced to undergo apoptosis by UVB as detected by the TUNEL method.[2] Furthermore, hyperplastic KC in untreated psoriatic plaques were induced by UVB to strongly express CD95L (FasL) which coincided temporally with the depletion of intra-epidermal T cells, suggesting that KC CD95L-T cell CD95 inter-action may result in the latter's demise.[8] Similarly, successful UVA radiation phototherapy in patients with atopic dermatitis has also been shown to result from UV radiation-induced apoptosis in skin-infiltrating TH cells leading to T cell depletion from eczematous skin.[9] This is likely to be mediated through the Fas/FasL system

Table 7.1   Mechanisms of action of current treatments used in psoriasis

Treatment	T cell/KC	Mechanism of Action
PUVA/UVB	T cells	Apoptosis via Fas/FasL pathway
CyA/FK506	T cells	Binds to immunophilin; inhibits calcineurin, translocation of NF-AT and IL-2/4 transcription
Vit. D analogues	KC	Nuclear: Vit.D/Vit.DR binds to VDRE of target genes
		Non-nuclear: intracellular signalling, incr. Ca^{++} influx
Vit. A analogues	T cells and KC	Nuclear: As Vit.D (differentiation)
	proliferation)	Indirect: blocks AP1 (inflammation/
Corticosteroids	T cells	Nuclear: As Vit.D
Methotrexate	T cells and KC	Apoptosis via Fas-independent pathway
	KC	Converts to polyglutamate; blocks DNA synthesis by inhibition of thymidine-monophosphate production
Dithranol	T cells and KC	Unknown

which can become activated in irradiated T cells as a consequence of singlet oxygen generation.[9]

7.1.2 *CyA and FK506*

The effective clearing of psoriatic lesions can be induced by systemic treatment with low doses of the immunosuppressant drugs CyA and FK506 (tacrolimus).[10-13] These drugs act primarily on activated T cells inhibiting their production of cytokines such as IL-2 and IFN-γ. Thus CyA-treated psoriatic lesions show a decrease in total

CD4$^+$ and CD8$^+$ T cells from both the epidermis and dermis. However, HLA-DR$^+$ CD4$^+$ T cells are present even after resolution.[14] In contrast, the latter group of cells is rapidly cleared from the epidermis after intralesional injection of CyA probably due to the increased local concentration of the drug.[15]

Although CyA and FK506 are structurally different (undecapeptide and macrolide, respectively), they have the same mode of action.[16] Each binds to an intracellular receptor or immunophilin which exist in many different isoforms; CyA binds to cyclophilin and FK506 to FK506-binding protein (FKBP). Interestingly, both types of immmunophilin have rotamase (peptidyl prolyl cis-trans isomerase) activity, but this function does not appear to be linked to the therapeutic benefits of these immunosuppressants. The two drug-protein complexes, cyclophilin-cyclosporin and FKBP-FK506, but not the drugs alone, bind to a protein phosphatase called calcineurin (Fig. 7.1).[17] Calcineurin is Ca^{++}- and calmodulin-dependent and consists of catalytic (A) and regulatory (B) subunits. The resultant inhibition of calcineurin activity results in a complete block in the translocation of the cytosolic component of the nuclear factor of activated T cells (NF-AT), resulting in a failure to activate the genes regulated by NF-AT such as IL-2 and IL-4. Calcineurin probably acts by dephosphorylating NF-AT which is a phosphoprotein in resting cells.[18]

In contrast, rapamycin (sirolimus), an analogue of FK506 which has also been proposed as a treatment for psoriasis, blocks T cell proliferation at a later stage during the G$_1$ to S phase progression.[19]

Clinical improvement with CyA is accompanied by the loss of ICAM-1 (CD54) expression on KC and decreased epidermal IL-8 and IL-1β mRNA levels.[20,21] However, the induction of expression of ICAM-1, IL-8 or gro-α mRNA by cultured KC in response to IL-1β or TNF-α plus IFN-γ were not inhibited by CyA, suggesting that CyA acts primarily through the blockade of T cells rather than through KC activation.[21,22]

FK506 has been shown to have no direct anti-proliferative effects on cultured human KC.[23] However, the drug causes a dose-dependent

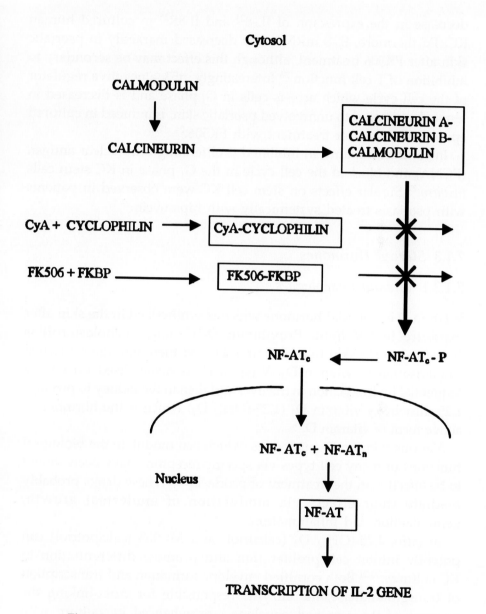

Fig. 7.1. Mechanism of action of CyA/FK506 on T cell function.

decrease in the expression of IL-8[24] and Il-8R[25] in cultured human KC. Furthermore, IL-8 mRNA was decreased markedly in psoriatic skin after FK506 treatment, although this effect may be secondary to inhibition of T cell function.[26] Interestingly, p53, a negative regulator of the cell cycle which arrests cells in G_1 phase and is decreased in lesional compared to uninvolved psoriatic skin, is induced in cultured epidermal cells after treatment with FK506.[24]

In contrast, rapamycin inhibited proliferating cell nuclear antigen (PCNA) and blocked the cell cycle in the G_1 phase in KC stem cells *in vitro*.[27] Similar effects on stem cell KC were observed in patients with psoriasis treated systemically with rapamycin.[27]

7.1.3 Steroid Hormones

7.1.3.1 Vitamin D analogues

Vitamin D is a steroid hormone which is synthesized in the skin after exposure to UV light. Provitamin D_3 (7-dehydrocholesterol) is converted in the skin to pre-vitamin D_3 and then undergoes thermal isomerisation to vitamin D_3. Vitamin D_3 is metabolised further by sequential hydroxylation in the liver and then in the kidney to produce 1,25 dihydroxy vitamin D_3 (1,25-$(OH)_2$ D_3) which is the hormonally active form of vitamin D.

Various vitamin D_3 analogues, which can modulate the biological functions of many cell types via specific receptors, have been shown to be effective in the treatment of psoriasis.[28,29] These drugs probably mediate their effects via modulation of epidermal growth, keratinization and inflammation.

In vitro, 1,25-$(OH)_2$ D_3 (calcitriol) and MC903 (calcipotriol) can potently inhibit cell proliferation and promote differentiation in KC cultures.[30,31] Both cornified envelope formation and transcription of transglutaminase, the enzyme responsible for cross-linking the proteins of the cornified envelope, are enhanced by culture with vitamin D analogues. The latter may also promote transcription and release of TGF-β, a cytokine with suppressive effects on KC proliferation, and conversely, *in vivo* inhibit expression of IL-6 which is stimulatory for KC growth.[32]

A significant increase in the expression of vitamin D receptors in basal and suprabasal layers of lesional psoriatic epidermis compared to that of normal skin has been reported, suggesting that the KC may be the primary target of the drugs in psoriasis.[33] However, Abe *et al.*[34] demonstrated resistance to the effects of calcitriol by cultured psoriatic KC from both lesional and uninvolved skin which required 100-fold more hormones than normal KC to inhibit their DNA synthesis.

Vitamin D analogues also exert a variety of effects on cells of the immune system. These include inhibition of the production of macrophage-derived cytokines such as IL-1α, IL-6 and TNF-α, probably via reduction of the half-life of specific mRNAs, and suppression of proliferation and cytokine production (IL-2 and IFN-γ) by activated T cells [reviewed in Ref. 35]. Furthermore, calcipotriol suppresses both the number and antigen-presenting function of LCs in normal human skin.[36]

Simultaneous assessment of inflammation and epidermal proliferation in psoriatic plaques during long-term treatment with calcipotriol revealed a significant decrease in polymorphonuclear (PMN) cells after one week of treatment followed by a reduction in numbers of actively cycling, Ki-67$^+$ epidermal cells after two weeks.[37] A decrease in T cells was not observed until after four weeks, at which time clinical improvement had already reached its maximum, and LCs tended to increase, in contrast to the findings in normal skin.[36] Thus, this and other studies,[38,39] suggest that vitamin D analogues predominately modulate KC function leaving the mononuclear cell infiltrate largely unaffected. Furthermore, a recent study has demonstrated that calcipotriene-induced clinical improvement of psoriasis was preceded by a (modest) increase in IL-10 and a concomitant decrease in IL-8 levels without significant changes in T cell numbers.[39] Compatible with this finding is the observation that calcipotriol and calcitriol induce IL-10R expression in human epidermal cells.[40]

Furthermore, the decrease in IL-8 could explain the early decrease in PMNs observed in the previous study.[37]

Two basic mechanisms are responsible for the action of vitamin D analogues; a nuclear mechanism involving the modification of gene transcription, and a non-nuclear mechanism involving signalling.

Active vitamin D_3 bound to highly specific nuclear receptors (VDRs) regulates gene transcription by binding to a specific sequence of DNA known as the vitamin D response element (VDRE). VDREs are present in the promotor region of target genes of active vitamin D_3. The vitamin D receptor has structural homology with known steroid receptors, such as glucocorticoid, thyroid and retinoic acid receptors, all of which belong to the nuclear receptor superfamily. The receptor is composed of three domains; one binds the steroid, a second binds DNA, and a third interacts with other members of the nuclear receptor superfamily. Indeed, the interaction of VDR with one of the members, retinoid-X receptor-alpha (RXR-α) enhances tight binding of VDR with VDRE (Fig. 7.2). Similarly, RXR-α also dimerises with thyroid receptors to increase binding. DNA response elements vary for different members of the nuclear receptor family. Furthermore, two classes of VDRE have been identified which are activated by VDR alone or by VDR-RXR-α heterodimers.

Active vitamin D_3 can also induce an increased influx of calcium into the cell via a non-nuclear mechanism. This has been demonstrated

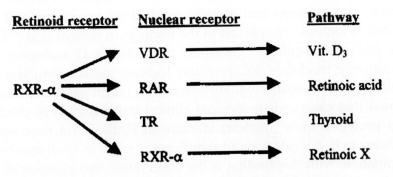

Fig. 7.2. Nuclear receptor superfamily interactions.

at physiological concentrations ($10^{-11} - 10^{-9}$M) in KC and occurs within 90 secs of the addition of the hormone to the culture medium.[41]

Modulation of intracellular signalling results from the nuclear effects and transmembrane calcium influx. Thus calcitriol enhances the production of inisitol triphosphate and 1,2 diacylglycerol and induces an increase of intracellular calcium. Vitamin D_3 also promotes the translocation of protein kinase C from the cytosol to the membrane.[42] Both protein kinase C and increased intracellular calcium concentration may act as mediators of the effects of vitamin D_3 on KC differentiation.

A large number of further vitamin D_3 analogues are currently being developed, some of which appear to be very potent T cell inhibitors of several orders of magnitude more active than CyA.[43] These new analogues will obviously be of potential interest in the treatment of psoriasis.

7.1.3.2 *Vitamin A analogues*

Vitamin A analogues (retinoids) have been used to treat psoriasis with variable success. One of the earliest drugs developed, isotretinoin (13-cis-retinoic acid), applied topically, failed to demonstrate any significant improvement in nine patients with CP psoriasis.[44] Second-generation retinoids, etrinate and its active metabolite acitretin, which are characterised by an aromatized β-oinone ring, are only used in severe and recalcitrant forms of psoriasis due to their attendant toxic side-effects. These oral retinoids are most effective in treating pustular and erythrodermic psoriasis, and less effective in treating CP psoriasis.[45] Tazarotene and tazarotenic acid are the first of a new generation of retinoids called acetylene retinoids which have been developed to be receptor selective.[46]

Retinoids have potent effects on proliferation, keratinization and differentiation of epidermal cells,[47] but their immunomodulating effects have appeared to be limited. However, in etretinate-treated psoriasis patients, an early decrease of serum IFN-γ to baseline levels before clinical improvement, and a 50–65% reduction in CD3[+], CD8[+] and CD25[+] T cell subsets accompanied by a loss in HLA-DR and ICAM-1 KC expression in lesional skin, have been reported.[48,49] The latter was accompanied by decreased KC proliferation and enhanced KC differentiation.[49] Topical tazarotene has also been shown to decrease inflammation in psoriatic skin.[46]

The actions of vitamin A analogues are, in common with those of vitamin D, exerted through receptors of the hormone receptor superfamily in the nucleus. Transcription of genes can be regulated by the activated retinoid-receptor complex either directly by binding to promotor regions of specific genes, or indirectly by blocking the transcriptional effects of other nuclear transcription factors such as AP1. AP1 is an oncogenic protein which regulates the transcription of genes associated with inflammation and proliferation such as IL-2. It is believed that the retinoid-induced effects on differentiation are mediated by the first mechanism, and the anti-proliferative and anti-inflammatory activities by the second.

Two families of retinoid nuclear receptors have been identified, retinoic acid receptors (RARs) and retinoid X receptors (RXRs), each of which include three subtypes (α, β and γ) encoded by distinct genes. RARγ is the predominant RAR species in human epidermis. RARs interact with RXRs for effective DNA binding and function. In addition, RXRs form heterodimers with other hormone receptors such as the vitamin D_3 receptors (Fig. 7.2).

7.1.3.3 Corticosteroids

Glucocorticosteroids are potent immunosuppressive drugs affecting T, B and macrophage function which are commonly used topically to treat mild to moderate psoriasis. These drugs inhibit proliferation and cytokine production by T lymphocytes and can, to varying extents, induce lymphocyte death (apoptosis).[50] Corticosteroids mediate their effects in the same way as the vitamin D and A analogues described above; that is, via binding to specific nuclear receptors. Steroid-induced resolution of of psoriatic plaques is preceded by the disappearance of T cells from the epidermis. Epidermal dendritic cells also disappear (or lose their markers), but this happens after the onset of clinical resolution.[51]

Topical glucocorticosteroids also inhibit proliferation and chemotaxis of fibroblasts and KC, *in vitro*, in a dose-dependent manner.[52]

7.1.4 *Methotrexate*

Methotrexate is a folate antagonist and potent antiproliferative agent that, after conversion to polyglutamate forms, blocks the synthesis of DNA by inhibiting thymidine monophosphate production. It also has a wide range of anti-inflammatory properties associated with the increased release of adenosine from different cell types.[53] However, unlike CyA, FK506 and glucocorticosteroids, methotrexate has no effect on cytokine release from T cells or monocytes.[54] Recently, the immunosuppressant properties of low-dose methotrexate, which is used in the treatment of severe psoriasis, have been shown to be mediated via selective apoptosis of activated peripheral blood T cells by a Fas-independent pathway.[55] Furthermore, methotrexate also induce apoptotic cell death in KC in an epidermal explant/dermal model *in vitro*.[56] Thus the beneficial effects of methotrexate in psoriasis may be mediated, at least in part, by the induction of apoptosis in both cell types.

7.1.5 *Dithranol*

Dithranol (anthralin) is a synthetic preparation related to a natural product, chrysarobin which has been used as an anti-psoriatic agent for more than 80 years. The drug appears to mediate its anti-psoriatic effects via inhibition of KC and lymphocyte proliferation.[57,58] Dithranol reduces the degree of acanthosis in psoriatic skin lesions by inducing a slow, steady decrease in epidermal thickness, but does not reduce cell renewal.[59] A major decrease in keratin 16 content and a virtually complete restoration of the filaggrin positive cell layer, but no reduction in transglutaminase- and involucrin-positive cells, has also been reported in psoriatic skin lesions treated with dithranol cream.[60] Furthermore, epidermal T cell numbers were decreased by about half, but this was subsequent to the onset of resolution.[51] In addition, total epidermal dendritic cell numbers were only marginally decreased, but the small HLA-DR+, CD1- subset had virtually disappeared.[51] The mode of action of dithranol remains to be elucidated.

7.2 Future Treatments

7.2.1 *Cell Surface Molecule-Directed*

Various cell surface molecules such as CD4, CD28/B7, TCR Vβ and MHC Class II, involved in the interaction between TCR, antigenic peptide and MHC-expressing antigen-presenting cells, are potential targets for intervention in the disease process. Two approaches are commonly used: administration of monoclonal antibodies (mAb) specific for molecules involved in antigen recognition and/or T cell activation, or the use of synthetic peptides (and proteins) to block MHC Class II-restricted activation of T cells or induce T cell tolerance. A third option is the blocking of homing receptors and/or their ligands which would inhibit the migration of T cells into the skin.

7.2.1.1 *CD4*

MAb to CD4 can be classified as depleting or non-depleting according to their cytotoxic effects on target cells. The non-depleting mAbs have the advantage of avoiding the induction of general immunosuppression and act in part by blockading the interaction between CD4 and TCR or MHC molecules.

As mentioned in Sec. 4.2, patients with severe psoriasis treated with a depleting murine anti-CD4 mAb showed rapid clinical improvement during the month after treatment but produced IgM

Table 7.2 **Novel immunological approaches to the treatment of psoriasis**

Target/Approach	Treatment
Cell surface molecules	
CD4	**Depleting/non-depleting mAbs**
Costim. molecules: LFA-1	**Humanized CD11a mAb**
CTLA-4	**CTLA-4Ig soluble fusion protein**
TCR	TCR Vβ mAb
	TCR antagonists, e.g. peptide analogues
MHC Class II	mAbs, antigenic peptides, MHC
	peptides.
Homing receptors	mAbs
Cytokines	
Admin. of cytokines	**IFN-γ, TNF-α, IL-10**, IL-4
Admin. of toxin-conjugated cytokines	**DAB$_{389}$IL-2**
TH$_1$ to TH$_2$: Inhibition of IL-12	IL-12 p40 homodimer (antagonist),
	cAMP-inducing drugs, modulation of
	IL-12-Rβ_2
Induction of IL-10	**Monomethyl fumarate**, cAMP-
	elevating drugs
Induction of regulatory T cells	
T cell vaccination	Attenuated autoimmune T cells
TCR peptides	**Vβ3 and Vβ13.1 peptides**
DNA encoding TCR Vβ	Injection of naked DNA
Oral tolerance	Oral or nasal immunisation with
	autoantigen
Apoptosis	Selective activation-induced cell death
	of pathogenic T cells or KC, e.g. anti-Fas
	mAb
Gene therapy	Transfer of genes for anti-inflammatory
	cytokines, pro-apoptotic proteins, TCR
	peptides or genes defective in disease
Novel anti-inflammatory/immuno-suppression drugs	Purine nucleoside phosphorylase
	inhibitors, e.g. BCX-34
	Topical ascomycin, e.g. **SDZ ASM 981**

*Treatments in bold indicate those tested in psoriatic patients.

and/or IgG antibodies against the therapeutic mAb.[61] More recently, non-depleting humanised anti-CD4 mAbs have been used to treat psoriasis in an open and unblinded, and double-blind, placebo-controlled study, respectively.[62,63] Clinical improvement was evident in most patients at the higher doses used and, in the latter study, patients with refractory psoriasis became easier to control with conventional agents after mAb therapy.[63] No patients developed significant changes in circulating CD4$^+$ T cell counts.

Short-course therapy with non-depleting anti-CD4 mAb may exert long-lasting effects since tolerance can be induced to antigens simultaneously injected with the mAb in animal models of autoimmune disease. However, no evidence for tolerance induction in human disease such as rheumatoid arthritis, in which several clinical trials have been carried out, has yet been observed.

7.2.1.2 *Costimulatory molecules*

In addition to ligation of the TCR by specific peptide, costimulatory molecules are necessary to fully activate T cells to proliferate, produce cytokines and exert cytolytic activity. A lack of one or more of these costimulatory signals can lead to T cell anergy, a state of unresponsiveness accompanied by lack of IL-2 production and proliferation. Thus, binding of the MHC Class II-bound peptide to the TCR on the T cell is accompanied by interactions between receptors and their ligands on T cells and APC, respectively: integrin LFA-1 (CD11a/CD18) and its counter-receptors ICAM-1/2/3; CD2 and LFA-3(CD58); CD40L and CD40; CD28/CTLA-4 and B7. Two of these costimulatory interactions are currently being targeted as a means of switching off the psoriatic process.

Anti-CD11a (LFA-1)

Recently, 31 patients with moderate to severe plaque psoriasis have been treated with a single infusion of humanised CD11a mAb at various doses.[64] CD11a, together with CD18, make up the LFA-1 molecule expressed on T cells which is important in T cell activation, cytotoxic T cell function and T cell adhesion to vascular endothelium and keratinocytes. Treatment with CD11a mAb resulted in down-modulation of surface CD11a expression by circulating T cells in a reversible, dose-dependent manner. In addition, a mean decrease in PASI score of 33% was observed in the majority of the patients at the higher dose. This was reflected in a decrease in epidermal CD3[+] and CD11a[+] T cells, decreased ICAM-1 expression by KC and endothelial cells, and epidermal thinning in lesional skin. These beneficial effects probably resulted from the inhibition of T cell activation and/or migration into the skin. However, reversible side-effects such as fever, chills and headaches were experienced which were moderate to severe at higher doses of the mAb.

Recently, an ICAM-1 anti-sense oligonucleotide was used in a placebo-controlled trial in the treatment of Crohn's disease, with beneficial effects observed.[65] The oligonucleotide specifically hybridises to a sequence in human ICAM-1 message resulting in the formation of a heterodimer. This is cleaved by RNase-H thus reducing ICAM-1 expression.[65]

CTLA-4Ig

CD28 and CTLA-4 (Cytolytic-T-Lymphocyte-associated Antigen-4), which are members of the same family and show extensive nucleotide homology are expressed on both CD4[+] and CD8[+] T cells.[66] However, CTLA-4, unlike CD28, is not found on resting T cells but is induced following signalling through the antigen-specific TCR.[67] Although both molecules bind to the B7/BB1 family of molecules expressed by APC, their functions appear to be opposing with CD28 acting as a costimulator of T cell activation whilst cross-linking of CTLA-4 results in decreased T cell proliferation due to down-regulated IL-2 production.[68] Thus blockade of CTLA-4/B7 interactions with mAbs or via deletion of the CTLA-4 gene promotes T cell expansion and cytokine production.

Human CTLA-4Ig, a soluble fusion protein of the extracellular domain of CTLA-4 with the constant region of human immunoglobulin-γ, effectively prevented human pancreatic islet graft rejection in mice, and prolonged heart allograft survival in rats.[69,70] Although the mechanisms involved remain to be clarified, the blocking of costimulation for IL-2 production, presumably by preventing CD28 interaction with B7/BB1, represents a novel approach to immune suppression which potentially could be useful for treating autoimmune diseases and preventing transplant rejections. Indeed a Phase 1 clinical trial of the use of CTLA-4Ig in psoriasis has been carried out.[71] Thirty seven patients with psoriasis were given four infusions of one of seven different dose levels ranging from 0.5 to 2.5 mg/kg. At the highest dose, five out of six patients showed virtual elimination of psoriatic features in skin lesions including significant reduction in intraepidermal T cells, epidermal thickness and Ki-67+ keratinocytes.[71]

7.2.1.3 TCR

mAb to TCR Vβ families

The clonal expansion of TCR Vβ2- and Vβ6- expressing CD4+ T cells, and of Vβ3- and Vβ13-expressing CD8+ T cells in psoriatic skin lesions (see Chap. 4) suggests that these cells may be pathogenic and, therefore, potential targets for selective immunosuppression by administration of specific anti-Vβ mAbs. Such an approach has been used successfully in animal models of autoimmune diseases such as experimental allergic encephalomyelitis (EAE).[72] However, optimisation of treatment required the use of a cocktail of mAbs directed against different parts of the Vβ sequence.[73] The heterogeneity of Vβ expression observed in some patients may limit the usefulness of this approach in psoriasis, but this remains to be tested.

TCR antagonists

Selective inhibition of T cell activation can also be induced by antigenic peptide analogues which act as TCR antagonists. It has recently been demonstrated that each amino acid in the antigenic peptide can influence both its binding to MHC on the APC, and the overall affinity of the MHC/peptide complex for the TCR.[74] The combination of positive and negative effects of individual amino acids in the antigenic peptide determines whether the resulting affinity of the MHC/peptide for the TCR is high enough to trigger TCR-dependent signalling.[75] Thus, providing the antigenic peptide specificity of the pathogenic T cell clones have been identified, peptides could potentially be designed which could bind to MHC, but fail to induce a T cell response. However, an autoimmune response is continually recruiting T cells with different specificities during progression of the disease, so-called epitope spreading. Thus antagonism of one population of autoreactive T cells could conceivably induce the emergence of T cells specific for alternative epitopes at an earlier stage of the disease. In addition, peptide analogues which antagonise one T cell clone may act as specific agonists of another which could result in exacerbation rather than amelioration of the disease.

This approach has yet to be applied to a human disease. Its possible use in psoriasis will obviously require identification of the pathogenic antigenic peptide(s) involved.

7.1.2.4 *MHC Class II*

Blockade of the MHC molecule involved in the presentation of the disease-inducing antigen (self or foreign) is another approach that has been employed in the prevention of experimental autoimmune diseases. This can be achieved with mAbs, antigenic peptides or with MHC peptides.

mAb directed against the MHC molecule, or the MHC Class II/ autoantigen peptide complex have been used to prevent the development of experimental autoimmune myasthenia gravis and

EAE, respectively in mice.[76,77] However, this approach could potentially cause general immunosuppression which might result in unwanted side-effects.

Peptides binding to the same MHC Class II molecule can compete with one another for presentation to T cells. This suggested a more selective means of inducing immunosuppression by blocking the binding sites of MHC Class II molecules associated with autoimmune diseases, thus preventing binding and presentation of the autoantigen to pathogenic T cells.

This approach has been successfully applied to the inhibition of EAE induction in mice using peptides unrelated to the autoantigen, but with high affinity for the relevant MHC Class II determinants.[78] This is relevant to human autoimmune disease in which the nature of the autoantigen, in most cases, is unknown. However, in the human disease, blocking peptides would have to displace the disease-inducing epitope already bound to the MHC Class II molecules rather than compete for initial binding as in the experimental situation. This would necessitate the blocking peptide to be of higher affinity than that of the autoantigenic peptide. In addition, long-term treatment of chronic autoimmune disease would require long-lived MHC saturation which has yet to be demonstrated *in vitro* or *vivo*.[79] Thus the feasibility of this approach in treating diseases such as psoriasis is doubtful.

A novel immunotherapeutic approach which may prove useful in human disease is the administration of synthetic peptides corresponding to short linear sequences of the HLA molecules themselves. These have inhibitory effects on human T cells *in vitro* and, furthermore, cause tolerance induction in a rat heterotopic heart transplant model.[80] The lymphocytes from these transplanted rats were shown to be anergic, that is, they specifically failed to respond when exposed to donor antigen. Both MHC Class I and MHC Class II peptides can be inhibitory but function by different mechanisms. Clinical trials of a MHC Class I peptide under the name "Allotrap" have revealed it to be non-toxic in humans.[80] Their ability to induce specific anergy and long-term tolerance would make these MHC peptides a promising means of inducing suppression in chronic diseases such as psoriasis.

7.2.1.5 *Homing receptors*

Prevention of T cell migration into the skin by blocking homing receptors (e.g. CLA) on T cells or their ligands on endothelial cells (e.g. E.selectin) using mAbs is another possible approach which has yet to be investigated in human disease.

7.2.2 *Cytokine-Directed*

Since cytokines play a key role in the pathogenesis of psoriasis, they represent an obvious target for immunotherapy. Thus, various cytokines have been administered to psoriatic patients in an attempt to switch the disease process off. Furthermore, conversion of the TH_1 type cytokine profile dominated by IFN-γ production to that of an anti-inflammatory IL-4-producing TH_2 phenotype would be predicted to be beneficial in psoriasis. This could be achieved by drugs or by IL-12 antagonists.

7.2.2.1 *IFN-γ*

Based upon the known anti-proliferative effects of IFN-γ on normal KC *in vitro*, 23 patients with CP psoriasis were treated with intra-muscular injection of different doses of human recombinant IFN-γ.[81] It was only in the group treated with doses of 0.25 mg/m^2 that there was any suggestion of improvement coincident with their therapy. However, only one of the ten patients given this dose inproved substantially. This lack of efficacy of IFN-γ treatment is, with hindsight, not surprising since it has been demonstrated by two groups that psoriatic KC have a decreased susceptibility to the inhibitory effects of this cytokine (see Sec. 6.2.2).

7.2.2.2 *TNF-α*

The effect of systemic administration of TNF-α was evaluated in three patients with extensive psoriasis.[82] Doses varied from 1×10^5 to $5 \times 10^5 \, U/m^2$ and each dose was administered for five day periods. Two of the patients showed improvement after the second course of treatment, and complete or significant improvement after the third course. The third patient who had more localised, less severe psoriasis did not, however, show any improvement with recombinant TNF-α treatment.

Two further cases of patients with severe psoriasis treated with recombinant TNF-α also showed complete or partial improvement in skin lesions.[83] However, significant toxicity, as suggested by fever and chills, was experienced by the treated patients.

The reasons for the beneficial effects of TNF-α administration in psoriasis are not known but may be related to the antiproliferative action of the cytokine on epidermal cells.

7.2.2.3 *IL-10*

IL-10 is very poorly expressed in psoriatic skin lesions, but an increase in IL-10 mRNA expression by PBMC has been observed in patients during established anti-psoriatic therapy, suggesting that IL-10 may have anti-psoriatic effects (see below).

On this basis, Asadullah *et al.*[84] performed a Phase II pilot trial with subcutaneous Il-10 administration (8 µg/kg/d) over 24 days in three patients. Clinical response to the administration of the cytokine was heterogenous, with a decrease in PASI score but not complete healing in each case. The treatment was well tolerated with no evidence of any adverse side effects. The skin lesions showed a decrease in epidermal thickness, parakeratosis and degree of infiltration. Immunosuppressive effects of the treatment included depressed monocytic HLA-DR expression, TNF-α and IL-12 secretion, decreased IL-12 plasma levels and reduced responsiveness to recall antigens. Furthermore, a shift towards a TH type 2 cytokine pattern with increased proportions of IL-4, IL-5 and IL-10 producing T cells and a selective increase in IgE serum levels was observed. Surprisingly, IL-10 administration also enhanced intracutaneous IL-10 mRNA expression.

7.2.2.4 IL-4

It has been demonstrated in animals that it is possible to induce antigen-specific CD4$^+$ T cells to produce IL-4 *in vivo*, by priming simultaneously with antigen and IL-4. Thus, therapeutic administration of IL-4 during exacerbation of an autoimmune disease should selectively induce IL-4 in activated, autoantigen-specific T cells whilst resting T cells specific for bacteria, for example, would retain their TH$_1$ response when specifically activated later.

Prevention of EAE in mice by innoculation of pathogenic MBP-specific TH cell lines, together with exogenous IL-4, was obtained only when MBP-specific TH$_2$ cells were generated by the therapy. Thus, this involved IL-4-induced immune deviation and was not merely secondary to the treatment with IL-4.[85]

IL-4-induced immune deviation is, therefore, a possible therapeutic approach for human TH$_1$-associated diseases such as psoriasis.

7.2.2.5 *Toxin-conjugated cytokines*

The potential use of immunotoxins in psoriasis has been demonstrated by the effectiveness of IL-2 fused to diptheria toxin DAB$_{389}$IL-2 (see Sec. 4.3).[86] This approach could be extended to other cytokines important in the pathogenesis of psoriasis such as IL-12, which would help to eliminate IFN-γ-producing TH$_1$ cells. However, problems such as rapid *in vivo* clearance, stimulation of the target cells when binding is insufficient for killing and competition by soluble ligands or receptors may limit the use of toxin-conjugated cytokines.

7.2.2.6 *Conversion of* TH_1 *to* TH_2 *cytokine profile*

Induction of TH_2 cell expansion in psoriasis could potentially inhibit the function of the disease-inducing TH_1 cells and thus switch off the disease. This conversion of a TH_1 to TH_2 type cytokine pattern could be achieved by the inhibition of IL-12 activity or conversely, induction of IL-10 production.

The IL-12 p40 homodimer, $p(40)_2$, binds to the IL-12R, but unlike the p75 heterodimer, does not transduce a signal, hence acting as an IL-12 antagonist. Administration of $p(40)_2$ has been used to treat EAE and prevent relapses in mice and could potentially be applied to a human TH_1 disease.[87]

In addition, several cAMP -inducing agents such as prostaglandin E_2 and adrenalin inhibit IL-12, but not IL-6 or IL-10 production. Furthermore, β-adrenergic compounds that also elevate intracellular cAMP act as potent and selective inhibitors of IL-12 production in humans, both *in vitro* and *in vivo*.[87]

Alteration of the TH_1/TH_2 balance may also be achieved by modulation of IL-12-dependent signalling. Two IL-12R subunits termed $β_1$ and $β_2$ have been identified which together give rise to high affinity binding sites. Whilst IL-12R$β_1$ transcripts are expressed in similar amounts in both TH_1 and TH_2 cells, IL-12R$β_2$ mRNA is selectively expressed in TH_1 lines only.[87] Since IL-12R$β_2$ contains the signalling component of the IL-12R, modulation of its expression on TH_1 cells represents another means by which the IFN-γ-dominated T cell response could be inhibited.

It has been shown *in vitro* that certain anti-psoriatic therapies such as UVB radiation and monomethyl fumarate induce an increase in IL-10 production in KC and monocytes, respectively.[88,89] Increased PBMC IL-10 mRNA expression has also been reported in psoriatic patients after treatment with UVB, or both PUVA and topical administration of dithranol and calcipotriol.[84] Furthermore, cAMP-elevating drugs such as iloprost and pentoxifylline, have been demonstrated to upregulate IL-10 production.[90] Interestingly, the latter has been shown to be effective in psoriasis.[91]

7.2.3 *Induction of Regulatory T Cells*

One mechanism by which autoimmune T cells may be restricted and prevented from expanding in the periphery involves an anti-clonotypic (anti-idiotypic) regulatory T cell network. Anti-clonotypic T cells recognise antigenic determinants (idiotopes) on the TCR and mediate protection mainly via cytotoxic effects. Thus, a lack of regulatory T cells required to maintain peripheral tolerance after an acute flare would allow an autoimmune response to be established and/or maintained.

Induction of regulatory T cells, therefore, represents a novel approach to the treatment of autoimmune diseases. This is being attempted using T cell vaccination or vaccination with TCR peptides or DNA encoding TCR Vβ regions, and by induction of oral tolerance.

7.2.3.1 *T cell vaccination*

The term T cell vaccination was first coined in 1981 to describe the use of attenuated autoimmune T cells as vaccines to prevent experimental autoimmune diseases.[92] The advantage of this approach is its specificity since it induces resistance to disease caused by pathogenic T cells of the same specificity as the T cell vaccine. As first demonstrated in the EAE animal model, the T cells must be activated (resting T cells have no effect) and attenuated by irradiation, hydrostatic pressure or chemical cross-linking, otherwise they induce disease rather than prevent it.[93] Alternatively, vaccination with unmodified autoimmune T cells can also be effective providing only a small number of cells is administered.[94]

Following the successful prevention of EAE and various other autoimmune diseases in animal models, the first experiments in humans were carried out in patients with multiple sclerosis.[95] T cell vaccination with inactivated MBP-reactive T cells resulted in depletion of circulating MBP-reactive T cells in a clonotypic-specific fashion. Furthermore, the immunity induced by T cell vaccination in these patients was long-lived.[95]

The feasibility of T cell vaccination in patients with rheumatoid arthritis and nickel allergy has also been investigated.[96,97] However, in rheumatoid arthritis patients, the vaccine was prepared from T cells of unknown specificity and thus modulation of a specific immune response could not be investigated. The same limitation would apply in patients with psoriasis. However, identification of the antigen-reactivity of disease-inducing T cells would make this a very attractive approach to a long-term resolution of this disease.

7.2.3.2 TCR peptides

TCR peptides unique to autoreactive T cells have also been used to induce resistance to autoimmune diseases such as EAE in animals. Resistance is mediated by peptide-specific T cells which down-regulate the activity of pathogenic T cells. In addition, anti-TCR peptide antibodies may also be involved.

The peptide-specific regulatory T cells are thought to be predomi-nately CD8+ T cells which recognise a homologue of the immunising peptide derived from processing of endogenous TCR proteins in the context of MHC Class I antigen on the surface of the pathogenic T cells. This would most likely result in direct cytolysis of the latter.

However, vaccination of MS patients with Vβ5.2 peptides from the complementarity-determining region -2 (CDR2), a hypervariable region of the TCR that interacts with MHC, boosted the frequency of CD4+ rather than CD8+ TCR peptide-reactive T cells.[98] The latter were predominately TH$_2$-like and directly inhibited MBP-specific TH$_1$ responses *in vitro* via release of IL-10. *In vivo*, the frequency of MBP-specific T cells was reduced and clinical progression of MS was prevented, without side-effects.[98]

The restricted TCR Vβ expression observed in psoriatic skin lesions makes TCR peptide vaccination a feasible therapeutic option in psoriasis. Indeed, a double-blind, Phase II clinical trial of a therapeutic vaccine consisting of Vβ3 and Vβ13.1 peptides has been carried out in patients with moderate to severe psoriasis by the Immune Response Corporation in California, USA, with promising results.[99]

7.2.3.3 DNA encoding TCR Vβ

Suppressive vaccination using naked DNA encoding a variable region of the TCR has also been reported in the EAE animal model.[100] Injection of Vβ8.2, which is expressed on pathogenic T cells that induce EAE, protected the mice from the disease and was accompanied by a reduction in the TH_1 cytokines IFN-γ and IL-2. In parallel, there was an increase in the production of IL-4, a TH_2 cytokine associated with suppression of the disease.

Targeting the TCR Vβ genes clonally expanded in psoriasis by DNA vaccination could be a useful therapeutic approach with the added advantage that the response to the target antigen may be shifted from a TH_1 to TH_2 cytokine response, thus helping to suppress bystander T cell responses.

7.2.3.4 Oral tolerance

Oral tolerance describes the state of systemic hyporesponsiveness which follows immunisation with a previously fed protein. This involves the stimulation of $CD8^+$ suppressor T cells, in an antigen-specific manner, to produce non-specific bystander suppression via the production of the inhibitory cytokine TGF-β.[101] However, although low doses of antigen favour active suppression, high doses induce deletion and anergy.[102] Administration of antigen via the nasal route appears to be equally effective and has the added advantage that smaller doses of antigen can be administered as compared to orally, perhaps due to the fact that there is less degradation of the proteins.

Suppression of autoimmunity by orally administered antigen appears to be a safe, feasible therapeutic option and is now being applied to the treatment of human diseases such as MS, RA, uveitis, diabetes and nickel allergy.[102,103]

The attraction of this approach is that it can suppress T cell responses to autoantigens without requiring exact knowledge of specificity and without general immunosuppression via bystander suppression. This provides a possible means of switching off the psoriatic disease process in which the (auto)antigen is unknown.

7.2.4 *Apoptosis-Based Therapy*

Selective induction of apoptosis or activation-induced cell death in pathogenic T cells has the potential for immunointervention in diseases such as psoriasis. As discussed in Sec. 7.1, conventional treatments for psoriasis such as PUVA and methotrexate induce apoptosis of T cells. Futhermore, psoriatic KC which express Fas, but do not appear to undergo apoptosis *in situ*, could be additional targets for therapy. Administration of anti-Fas antibody into the arthritic joint space of HTVL-1 *tax* transgenic mice improved their arthritis due to the elimination of Fas⁺ cells.[104] Such an approach could induce apoptosis of both activated T cells and epidermal cells in psoriatic skin lesions inducing resolution.

7.2.5 *Gene Therapy*

Knowledge of the identity of the genes which confer predisposition for the development of psoriasis is now within reach (see Sec. 1.2). Thus, gene therapy for psoriasis could become a reality in the forsee-able future. This could include, for example, administration of a gene encoding a protein that is defective in psoriasis. However, since it is clear that there are several genes implicated in disease susceptibility, the combination of which may vary between ethnic groups or even between families, substituting only one defective gene is unlikely to be curative.

Presently, a more realistic goal is the transfer of genes encoding proteins (or anti-sense RNA to block gene expression) which have the potential to improve psoriasis and which traditionally are administered orally or by injection. The advantage of this approach over drug therapy would be increased efficiency of delivery, sustained *in situ* production of the gene products eliminating the need for frequent readministration and specific localisation of the protein to the site of disease activity.

Keratinocytes have been shown to be suitable target cells for gene therapy. The transduction of a human IL-10 gene into the skin of hairless rats by the naked DNA injection method has demonstrated not only local expression of IL-10 mRNA and protein, but also circulating cytokine which could potentially exert biological effects at distant areas of the skin.[105] These findings have obvious implications for the treatment of psoriasis; genes coding for anti-inflammatory cytokines (IL-4, IL-10), pro-apoptotic proteins (Fas, FasL, bax, bak) or TCR peptides which induce regulatory T cells could potentially be introduced in this way to induce the resolution of skin lesions.

7.2.6 *Purine Nucleoside Phosphorylase Inhibitors/Ascomycins*

Novel anti-inflammatory and immunosuppressive drugs are continually being developed. One example is a purine nucleoside inhibitor BCX-34 which inhibits T cell proliferation (without suppression of IL-2 production) and is accompanied by the accumulation of intracellular dGTP with an associated reduction in GTP.[106] This inhibitor is currently being proposed as a novel therapy for psoriasis.[107]

Results of studies of the topical treatment of allergic contact dermatitis in pigs with the novel anti-inflammatory drug SDZ ASM 981, an ascomycin macrolactam derivative suggested that it might be effective in the topical treatment of skin disease in man.[108] SDZ ASM 981 inhibits T cell activation by inhibiting T cell proliferation and antigen-specific activation; production of both TH_1 and TH_2 type cytokines are inhibited. This new drug has proved effective in the treatment of atopic dermatitis[109] and clearing of psoriatic lesions has also been reported after topical application of 1% SDZ ASM 981 ointment under occlusion for 14 days.[109]

References

1. Baker B.S. *et al. Clin.Exp.Immunol.* **61** (1985), 526–534.
2. Krueger J.G. *et al. J.Exp.Med.* **182** (1995), 2057–2068.
3. Friedmann P. *Br.J.Dermatol.* **105** (1981), 219–221.
4. Aberer W. *et al. J.Invest.Dermatol.* **76** (1981), 202–210.
5. Olaniran A.K. *et al. Arch.Dermatol.Res.* **288** (1996), 421–425.
6. Oxholm A., Oxholm P., Staberg B., Bendtzen K. *Acta Dermatol.Venereol. (Stockh)* **69** (1989), 195–199.
7. Watts P., Stables G.S., Akhurst R.J., Mackie R.M. *Br.J.Dermatol.* **131** (1994), 64–71.
8. Gutierrez-Steil C. *et al. J.Clin.Invest.* **101** (1998), 33–39.
9. Morita A. *et al. J.Exp.Med.* **186** (1997), 1763–1768.
10. Griffiths C.E.M. *et al. Br.J.Med.* **293** (1986), 731–732.
11. Ellis C.N. *et al. J.Am.Med.Assoc.* **256** (1986), 3110–3116.
12. Van Joost T.H. *et al. Br.J.Dermatol.* **114** (1986), 615–620.
13. Jegasothy B.V. *et al. Arch.Dermatol.* **128** (1992), 781–785.
14. Baker B.S. *et al. Br.J.Dermatol.* **116** (1987), 503–510.
15. Baker B.S. *et al. Br.J.Dermatol.* **120** (1989), 207–213.
16. Liu J. *Immunol.Today* **14** (1993), 290–295.
17. Liu J. *et al. Cell* **66** (1991), 807–815.
18. McCaffrey P.G., Perrino B.A., Soderling T.R., Rao A. *J.Biol.Chem.* **268** (1993), 3747–3752.
19. Dumont F.J. *et al. J.Immunol.* **144** (1990), 251–258.
20. Horrocks C., Duncan J.I., Oliver A.M., Thomson A.W. *Clin.Exp.Immunol.* **84** (1991), 157–162.
21. Elder J.T. *et al. J.Invest.Dermatol.* **101** (1993), 761–766.
22. Kojima T. *et al. J.Invest.Dermatol.* **101** (1993), 767–772.
23. Duncan J.I. *J.Invest.Dermatol.* **102** (1994), 84–88.
24. Michel G. *et al. Biochem.Pharmacol.* **51** (1996), 1315–1320.
25. Schulz B.S. *et al. J.Immunol.* **151** (1993), 4399–4406.
26. Lemster B.H. *et al. Clin.Exp.Immunol.* **99** (1995), 148–154.
27. Javier A.F. *et al. J.Clin.Invest.* **99** (1997), 2094–2099.
28. Morimoto S. *et al. Br.J.Dermatol.* **115** (1986), 421–429.
29. Kragballe K., Beck H.I., Sogaard H. *Br.J.Dermatol.* **119** (1988), 223–230.
30. Smith E.L., Walworth N.C., Holick M.F. *J.Invest.Dermatol.* **86** (1986), 709–714.

31. Kragballe K., Wildfang I.L. *Arch.Dermatol.Res.* **282** (1990), 164–167.
32. Oxholm A., Oxholm P., Staberg B., Bendtzen K. *Acta Dermatol.Venereol. (Stockh)* **69** (1989), 385–390.
33. Milde P. *et al. J.Invest.Dermatol.* **97** (1991), 230–239.
34. Abe J., Kando S., Nishii Y., Kuroki T. *J.Clin.Endocrinol.Metab.* **68** (1989), 851–854.
35. Muller K. and Bendtzen K. *J.Invest.Dermatol.Symp.Proc.* **1** (1996), 68–71.
36. Dam T.N., Moller B., Hindkjaer J., Kragballe K. *J.Invest.Dermatol.Symp. Proc.* **1** (1996), 72–77.
37. De Jong E.M.G.J. and Van de Kerkof P.C.M. *Br.J.Dermatol.* **124** (1991), 221–229.
38. Verburgh C.A. and Niebaer C. *J.Invest.Dermatol.* **93** (1989), 310 (Abstract).
39. Kang S. *et al. Br.J.Dermatol.* **138** (1998), 77–83.
40. Michel G. *et al. Imflamm.Res.* **46** (1997), 32–34.
41. Bittiner B., Bleehen S.S., MacNeil S. *Br.J.Dermatol.* **124** (1991), 230–235.
42. Yada Y., Ozeki T., Meguro S. *Biochem.Biophys.Res.Commun.* **163** (1989), 1517–1522.
43. Binderup L. *et al. Biochem.Pharmacol.* **42** (1991), 1569–1575.
44. Bischoff R. *et al. Clin.Exp.Dermatol.* **17** (1992), 9–12.
45. Gollnick H. and Orfanos C.E. In *Psoriasis*, Reonigh H.H. Jr and Maibach H.I. (eds), Dekker, New York (1991), pp. 725–748.
46. Chandraratna R.A.S. *Br.J.Dermatol.* **135** (1996), 18–25.
47. Stadler R., Muller M., Detmar M., Orfanos C.E. *Dermatologica* **175, Suppl I** (1987), 45–55.
48. Shiohara T., Imanishi K., Sagawa Y., Nagashima M. *J.Am.Acad.Dermatol.* **27** (1992), 568–574.
49. Gottlieb S. *et al. J.Cutan.Pathol.* **23** (1996), 404–418.
50. Perrin-Wolff M. *et al. Biochem.Pharmacol.* **50** (1995), 103–110.
51. Baker B.S. *et al. Scand.J.Immunol.* **22** (1985), 471–477.
52. Wach F. *et al. Skin Pharmacol.Appl.Skin Physiol.* **11** (1998), 43–51.
53. Cronstein B.N., Eberle M.A., Gruber H.E., Levin R.I. *Proc.Natl.Acad.Sci. (USA)* **88** (1991), 2441–2445.
54. Schmidt J. *et al. Immunopharmacol.* **27** (1994), 173–179.
55. Genestier L. *et al. J.Clin.Invest.* **102** (1998), 322–328.
56. Heenen M., Laporte M., Noel J.C., de Graef C. *Arch.Dermatol.Res.* **290** (1998), 240–245.

57. Mahrle G., Bonnekoh B., Wevers A., Hegemann L. *Acta Dermatol.Venereol. (Stockh)* **186** (1994), 83–84.

58. Gaudin D., Greggs R.S., Yielding K.L. *Biochem.Biophys.Res.Commun.* **48** (1972), 945–949.

59. Bacharach-Buhles M., Rochling A., el Gammal S., Altmeyer P. *Acta Dermatol.Venereol. (Stockh)* **76** (1996), 190–193.

60. Van der Vleuten C.J., de Jong E.M., van de Kerkhof P.C. *Clin.Exp. Dermatol.* **21** (1996), 409–414.

61. Morel P. *et al. J.Autoimmun.* **5** (1992), 465–477.

62. Gottlieb A.B. *et al. J.Invest.Dermatol.* **110** (1998), 678 (Abstract).

63. Isaacs J.D. *et al. Clin.Exp.Immunol.* **110** (1997), 158–166.

64. Gottlieb A. *et al. J.Invest.Dermatol.* **110** (1998), 679 (Abstract).

65. Yacyshyn B.R. *et al. Gastroenterol.* **114** (1998), 1133–1142.

66. Harper K. *et al. J.Immunol.* **147** (1991), 1037–1044.

67. Lindsten T. *et al. J.Immunol.* **151** (1993), 3489–3499.

68. Krummel M.F. and Allison J.P. *J.Exp.Med.* **183** (1996), 2533–2540.

69. Lenschow D.J. *et al. Science* **257** (1992), 789–792.

70. Turka L.A. *et al. Proc.Natl.Acad.Sci. (USA)* **89** (1992) 11102–11105.

71. Krueger J.G. *et al. J.Invest.Dermatol.* **108** (1997), 555 (Abstract).

72. Acha-Orbea H. *et al. Cell* **54** (1988), 263–273.

73. Sakai K. *et al. Proc.Natl.Acad.Sci. (USA)* **85** (1988), 8608–8612.

74. Hemmer B. *et al. J.Immunol.* **160** (1998), 3631–3636.

75. Hemmer B. *et al. J.Exp.Med.* **185** (1997), 1651–1659.

76. Waldor M.K., Sriram S., McDevitt H.O., Steinman L. *Proc.Natl.Acad.Sci. (USA)* **80** (1983), 2713–2717.

77. Aharoni R., Teitelbaum D., Arnan R., Puri J. *Nature* **351** (1991), 147–150.

78. Lamont A.G. *et al. J.Immunol.* **145** (1990), 1687–1693.

79. Ishioka G.Y. *et al. J.Immunol.* **152** (1994), 4310–4319.

80. Krensky A.M. and Clayberger C. *Clin.Immunol.Immunopathol.* **75** (1995), 112–116.

81. Morhenn V.B. *et al. Arch.Dermatol.* **123** (1987), 1633–1637.

82. Takematsu H. *et al. Br.J.Dermatol.* **124** (1991), 209–210.

83. Creaven P.J. and Stall H.L. *J.Am.Acad.Dermatol.* **24** (1991), 735–737.

84. Asadullah K. *et al. J.Clin.Invest.* **101** (1998), 783–794.

85. Racke M.K. *et al. J.Exp.Med.* **180** (1994), 1961–1966.

86. Gottlieb S.L. *et al. Nat.Med.* **1** (1995), 442–447.

87. Adorini L. and Sinigaglia F. *Immunol.Today* **18** (1997), 209–211.

88. Enk C.D., Sredni D., Blauvelt A., Katz S.I. *J.Immunol.* **154** (1995), 4851–4856.
89. Asadullah K. *et al. Arch.Dermatol.Res.* **289** (1997), 623–630.
90. Platzer C. *et al. Int.Immunol.* **7** (1995), 517–523.
91. Gilhar A. *et al. Acta Dermatol.Venereol. (Stockh)* **76** (1996), 437–441.
92. Ben-Nun A., Wekerle H., Cohen I.R. *Nature* **292** (1981), 60–61.
93. Cohen I.R. *Immunol.Rev.* **94** (1986), 5–21.
94. Segel L.A., Jager E., Elias D., Cohen I.R. *Immunol.Today* **80** (1995), 80–84.
95. Zhang J., Stinissen P., Medaer R., Raus J. *J.Mol.Med.* **74** (1996), 653–662.
96. Van Laar J.M. *et al. J.Autoimmun.* **6** (1993), 159–167.
97. Dolhain R.J.E.M. *et al. J.Invest.Dermatol.* **105** (1995), 143–144.
98. Vandenbark A.A. *et al. Nat.Med.* **2** (1996), 1109–1115.
99. Gottlieb A.B. *Arch.Dermatol.* **133** (1997), 781–782.
100. Waisman A. *et al. Nat.Med.* **2** (1996), 899–905.
101. Miller A. *et al. Proc.Natl.Acad.Sci (USA)* **89** (1992), 421–425.
102. Weiner H.L. *Immunol.Today* **18** (1997), 335–343.
103. Bagot M. *et al. Eur.J.Dermatol.* **5** (1995), 614–617.
104. Fujisawa K. *et al. J.Clin.Invest.* **98** (1996), 271–278.
105. Meng X. *et al. J.Clin.Invest.* **101** (1998), 1462–1467.
106. Bantia S., Montgomery J.A., Johnson H.G., Walsh G.M. *Immunopharmacol.* **35** (1996), 53–63.
107. Walsh G.M. *et al.* In *Psoriasis*, Roenigh H.H. and Maibach H.I. (eds), Marcel Dekker, New York (1998).
108. Meingasser J.G. *et al. Br.J.Dermatol.* **137** (1997), 568–576.
109. van Leent E.J.M. *et al. Arch.Dermatol.* **134** (1998), 805–809.

Model for the Immunopathogenesis of Psoriasis

The linkage between HLA antigens and psoriasis, the persistence of the disease throughout life once it has manifested suggesting the existence of a "memory", and the spontaneous exacerbations and remissions of disease activity all strongly support an ongoing immune response in psoriasis.

In 1984, it was demonstrated that the eruption of acute psoriatic lesions coincided with the epidermal influx and activation of CD4[+] T cells, whereas disease resolution was associated with the recruitment of CD8[+] T cells.[1] On the basis of these and other findings, it was postulated that psoriasis is a disease of abnormal KC proliferation induced by T cells.[2] The evidence in support of this paradigm is now extensive (see Chap. 4), and the latter has become widely accepted amongst dermatologists investigating the pathogenic mechanisms of psoriasis.

8.1 Outline of Proposed Model

Initiation, and maintenance of psoriasis requires the presentation of antigen (superantigen/bacterial/viral/autoantigen) by MHC Class II-positive LC to CD4[+] T cells in the epidermis (Fig. 8.1; Table 8.1). This leads to the release by activated CD4[+] T cells of cytokines which stimulate KC proliferation, and the expression of adhesion molecules by KC and endothelial cells. KC, in turn, are stimulated to secrete a variety of cytokines which can act in an autocrine and/or paracrine

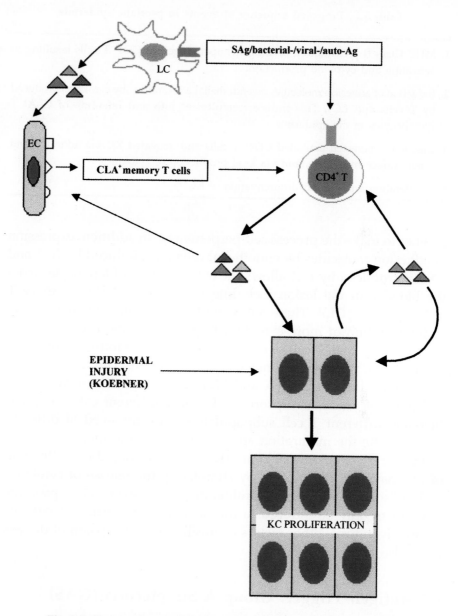

Fig. 8.1. Proposed model for the immunopathogenesis of psoriasis.

Table 8.1   Proposed sequence of events in psoriatic epidermis

1. MHC Class II presentation of antigen/superantigen to CD4$^+$ T cells resulting in activation and cytokine production.

2. Induction of adhesion molecules on endothelial cells and KC by cytokines produced by T cells and LCs. This induces recruitment into and retention of CLA$^+$ T lymphocytes in the epidermis.

3. Interaction between activated CD4$^+$ T cells and activated KC via adhesion and other surface molecules, and via local production of cytokines.

4. Proliferation and altered differentiation of KC.

manner to make the process self-perpetuating. In addition, expression of adhesion molecules by endothelial cells (also induced by IL-1 and TNF-α produced by LC) allows the extravasation of leukocytes from the blood into the lesion including skin-homing CD4$^+$ memory T cells expressing CLA. These cells would also become activated leading to the secretion of more cytokines to perpetuate the process.

It is likely that T cell-derived cytokines are required throughout the psoriatic process and not just for initiation. This is suggested by the effectiveness of CyA and FK506, and anti-CD4 mAbs in the treatment of established psoriasis. Possibly different cytokines, and therefore different T cell subpopulations, are involved at different stages of the the maturation and resolution of a lesion.

In the case of epidermal injury (Koebner reaction), direct activation of KC may start the process by stimulating the release of cytokines and subsequent epidermal proliferation. However, since psoriatic lesions can only be induced in this way in a proportion of patients at any given time, other factors controlling the expression of disease must also be involved.

8.2 Antigen Trigger: Group A Streptococci (GAS)

Although many environmental factors have been implicated, throat infection with GAS is the only external trigger convincingly asociated with initiation and exacerbation of psoriasis (see Chap. 5). Preceding streptococcal infection can be demonstrated in the majority of patients with guttate psoriasis, and also in many patients with exacerbation of CP psoriasis. The proposed model has therefore been based upon streptococci as the antigen trigger. This is not meant to imply that this applies to all patients with psoriasis. The involvement of other organisms as potential inducing antigens in psoriasis is discussed in Sec. 8.6.

There is evidence to suggest that both streptococcal pyrogenic exotoxins, which act as potent superantigens, and cell wall/membrane proteins expressed by GAS may be involved in the initiation and maintenance of the psoriatic process, respectively.

8.2.1 *Streptococcal Superantigens Induce Psoriasis*

Clinical experience of scarlet fever indicates that streptococcal pyrogenic exotoxins can become localised in the skin as a result of streptococcal throat infections as shown by the prevention or resolution of the skin rash by intradermal injection of antisera to the toxins (the Schultz-Charlton test).

The first indication that superantigens (SAg) may be involved in the pathogenesis of psoriasis came from the finding that Vβ2⁺ T cells were polyclonally expanded in acute guttate lesions.[3,4] In addition, all the streptococcal isolates from the guttate patients secreted SPE-C,[4] a SAg which is known to stimulate Vβ2⁺ T cells. In addition, other Vβ families found to be over-represented in psoriatic lesions (Vβ5.1, Vβ8 and Vβ12) are included in the repertoire of T cell subpopulations stimulated by streptococcal SAg. However, the presence of streptococcal toxins in acute psoriatic lesions has yet to be demonstrated.

To determine if a SAg could induce psoriasis, the staphylococcal exfoliative toxin was injected intradermally into uninvolved psoriatic skin grafted onto SCID mice. This resulted in an inflammation that exhibited some of the features of psoriasis.[5] Furthermore, peritoneal injection of SAg-stimulated T cells resulted in the homing of CLA[+] T cells to graft epidermis.[5] The ability of bacterial toxins to induce the expression of skin-homing receptors on T cells is, therefore, likely to be of relevance to the psoriatic process.[6]

8.2.2 *Antigen-Specific Response*

Thus it is possible that guttate psoriasis may be induced by SAg-activated T cells in a similar manner to that observed in scarlet fever. However, in scarlet fever, the skin rash fades within two weeks. In contrast, guttate psoriatic skin lesions, which also appear a few days after the throat infection, usully persist for 8–12 weeks, and psoriatic plaques often persist for many years. Therefore, additional factors are likely to be involved in psoriasis. This may include an antigen-specific T cell response directed to foreign and/or autoantigens.

In contrast to the early guttate lesions, analysis of Vβ gene usage in CP lesions revealed elevated expression of Vβ2 and Vβ6 (epi)dermal T cells (presumably CD4[+] T cells)[7] and of Vβ3 and Vβ13.1 epidermal CD8[+] T cells.[8,9] Furthermore, the increased expression was usually associated with a restricted number of dominant clones infiltrating the psoriatic lesions.[7-9] These findings strongly suggested that these dominant clones had been expanded *in situ* in response to an antigen or antigens in the skin. For the epidermal CD8[+] T cells, no consensus CDR3 (Vβ-Dβ-Jβ) motifs were present in most patients suggesting that different epidermal (auto)antigenic epitopes were presented in different patients. Alternatively, if a single epitope was responsible, the Vα chain associated with the Vβ chain, or possibly the Vβ region itself, may be crucial in antigen reactivity. In contrast, certain conserved junctional motifs of Vβ2 and/or Vβ6 and certain other Vβ families were found to be shared by different patients.[7,10] Furthermore, three motifs present in the CDR3 region of the dominant Vβ6 TCR of three of the patients were also detected amongst the the clonally expanded epidermal CD8[+] T cells expressing Vβ3 or Vβ13.1/3 TCR genes.[7,8] Conserved junctional CDR3 motifs joined to different Vβ segments have been reported in T cell clones specific for the same peptide/MHC complex.[10] It is therefore conceivable that the oligoclonal CD4[+] and CD8[+] T cell subpopulations present in the (epi)dermis and epidermis, respectively, could in some cases recognise the same antigenic epitope(s).

Thus, there is convincing evidence in CP lesions of an antigen-specific T cell response. The persistence of the same dominant clones in individual patients over several months suggests that this immune response is maintained against the same antigen by the same clonal T cell subpopulations.[7–9] The identity of the antigen(s) recognised is, as yet, unknown.

Evidence of an antigen-specific response in developed guttate psoriatic lesions has been obtained by culturing TCL from lesional skin of five patients in the presence of GAS.[11] Stable T cell clones isolated from one of the TCL recognised GAS in a HLA-DR-restricted manner indicating classical rather than SAg-mediated T cell activation.[11] These T cell clones were subsequently shown to be M12 cell wall protein-reactive (Baker B.S. *et al.*, unpublished observations). Interestingly, an over-representation of Vβ2 TCR was observed in five out of seven TCL obtained from guttate psoriatic lesions, while one TCL showed an increase in Vβ5.1 and Vβ12.[12] T cell reactivity to streptococcal cell wall and, particularly cell membrane proteins, has also been demonstrated by TCL isolated from CP patients. Consistent restricted TCR Vβ expression was not, however, observed in these streptococcal antigen-reactive CP TCL (Baker B.S. *et al.*, unpublished observations).

8.2.3 *Perpetuation of the Psoriatic Process*

Three pathways are proposed for the perpetuation of the psoriatic process subsequent to SAg activation of Vβ2[+] T cells (Fig. 8.2).

Activation of a streptococcal antigen-reactive Vβ2[+] T cell subset by (1) streptococcal antigen persisting in the skin or (2) by a cross-reactive skin determinant. (3) Stimulation by a skin determinant of an auto-reactive Vβ2[+] T cell subset expanded by the SAg over a threshold level.

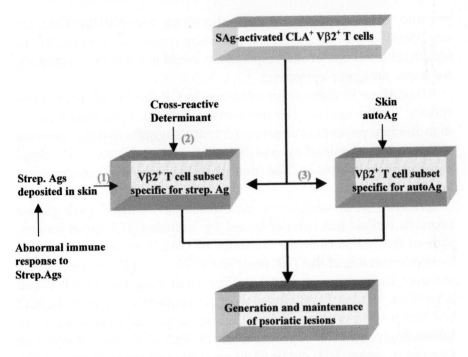

Fig. 8.2. Proposed pathways for the perpetuation of the psoriatic process.

Superantigenic activation of CLA$^+$ V$\beta2^+$ T cells by streptococcal toxins in psoriatic skin would cause proliferation and expansion of the T cell subset, and of any other T cells expressing appropriate TCR Vβ genes, regardless of their fine antigen specificity. However, the recognition of SAgs by T cells can lead subsequently to anergy and cell death. Thus, maintenance of the psoriatic process would require that a subset of the SAg-activated T cells is rescued from deletion; this is achieved by activation by a streptococcal or auto-antigen.

8.2.3.1 *Pathway 1*

Altered cell-mediated immunity to GAS has been demonstrated both *in vivo* and *in vitro* in individuals with guttate or CP psoriasis.

Futhermore, guttate psoriasis patients exhibited a significantly increased humoral response to streptococcal antigens compared to normal controls (see Secs. 5.5 and 5.6). Thus, it appears that at least some psoriatic patients may have an inherited abnormality of the immune system with respect to streptococcal antigens which may involve altered antigen processing or presentation by macrophages/dendritic cells and/or abnormal T lymphocyte responses. This could lead to inefficient clearing of the organism from the body and deposition of either non-viable streptococcal antigens, or perhaps even persistent slow-growing bacteria in the skin.

Detection of the presence of streptococci in psoriatic skin has proved problematic since mAb specific for GAS cross-react with various determinants in both normal and psoriatic skin.[13] Futhermore, PCR analysis of bacterial DNA in lesional skin would not discriminate between the causative agent and any organisms that had subsequently infected the lesional skin.

It has been demonstrated in patients with reactive arthritis that bacterial antigens can persist for years in the joints. It is therefore not inconceivable that a similar scenario could exist in the skin of patients with psoriasis. If so, this would make psoriasis a disease of chronic infection and would eliminate the need to invoke autoantigens as stimuli for T cell activation.

8.2.3.2 Pathway 2

The M proteins, the major virulence factors of GAS, share sequence homologies with mammalian fibrillar proteins from various organs including the skin. For example, the sequenced M6 protein has been shown to have a high degree of homology with type 1 50 kDa keratin (K14); this homology exists between various M serotypes and keratins.[12,14] K14 is present in increased quantities and preferentially expressed in psoriatic skin.[15] Both proteins have repeated segments of 7 AAs with only a single AA difference, an arrangement that might be expected to give rise to cross-reactivity at the T cell level because the latter recognise segments of primary (peptide) structure. Futhermore, it has been suggested that the predisposition to psoriasis may include a special allelic variant or a mutation of one or more of the keratin genes that are preferentially expressed by hyperproliferating KC.[12] Such "psoriatic" keratin could contain an epitope that is particularly cross-reactive with M protein, perhaps because it is more efficiently presented. Furthermore, upregulation of expression of this keratin may be induced by cytokines produced by SAg- or antigen-stimulated T cells.

However, other potentially M protein cross-reactive molecules exist in lesional psoriatic skin, such as heat shock proteins and the KC differentiation marker involucrin, which should also be considered as possible candidates for the role of psoriatic autoantigen.

What evidence is there to support this theory? Sigmundsdottir et al.[16] have shown that the IFN-γ responses of peripheral blood T cells from patients with active psoriasis were significantly higher to M6 peptides sharing 5–6 of their 20 AAs with keratin, than those of healthy or atopic dermatitis controls. These responses were abolished after the successful treatment of the psoriatic patients. However, it was not formally proven that the epitope(s) recognised within each M6 peptide included the AAs common to keratin. Further studies of T cell responses to keratin peptides by the same group have shown that the strongest and most frequent IFN-γ response by circulating psoriatic T cells was to a peptide from K17, which is one of the keratins upregulated in psoriasis.[17] This peptide shared 6 AA with M protein and was the only keratin peptide tested that induced a significantly higher response in psoriatic patients than healthy controls. Furthermore, the response was higher than to the corresponding M peptide.

However, the ability of M protein-reactive T cells to cross-react with proteins of a similar structure may not, in itself, be sufficient to cause disease. M peptide-specific TCL generated from a normal donor with no history of rheumatic fever was shown to respond, not only to the stimulating peptide, but to myosin peptides, porcine heart myosin and human rheumatic mitral valve.[18] In addition, the presence of M-specific T cells in psoriatic skin lesions has proved difficult to demonstrate with certainty, except for a single guttate TCL (see Sec. 8.2.2). Thus the relevance of these findings in peripheral blood to the psoriatic process in the skin has yet to be established.

8.2.3.3 Pathway 3

An extensive repertoire of self-antigens exists that are not normally accessible to the immune system because APC do not process them and present them efficiently for recognition by T cells. These self-antigens are referred to as cryptic. Potentially autoreactive but silent T cells specific for cryptic epitopes are not deleted in the thymus nor are they tolerized (unresponsive or anergic) in the periphery because the self-antigens they recognise are not normally presented at levels that can be recognised. Thus these autoreactive T cells, which are normal constituents of the T cell repertoire, are considered to be "ignorant" since they are unaware of the presence of their specific antigen.

Stimulation by streptococcal SAgs may trigger autoimmunity in psoriasis by expanding a subpopulation of ignorant autoreactive $V\beta2^+$ T cells, or by lowering the threshold level of a normally cryptic self-antigen that is required for autoreactive T cell stimulation. In addition, there are a variety of other mechanisms by which streptococcal infection could alter antigen processing and presentation leading to activation of previously ignorant autoreactive T cells. For example, activation of APC by microbial products such as LPS or by bacterial DNA can induce antigen-specific differentiation of autoreactive effector cells via the production of IL-12.[19] Of relevance to this finding is the increased levels of IL-12 that have been demonstrated in psoriatic lesions.[20]

This model would not require the autoantigen to be cross-reactive with a streptococcal antigen. It would however be compatible with that concept.

8.3 CD4⁺ T Lymphocyte/KC Interaction

8.3.1 *Surface Molecules*

Activated CD4⁺ T cells produce IFN-γ and TNF-α which together induce the expression of ICAM-1 by KC resulting in cell to cell contact between the two cell types via LFA-1/ICAM-1 interaction (Fig. 8.3). This interaction has been shown to be crucial in the presentation of SAg by MHC Class II-positive KC to T cells.[21] However, MHC Class II expression by psoriatic KC is observed only infrequently. It is therefore unlikely that presentation of antigen by KC to CD4⁺ T cells plays an important role in the pathogenic process.

IFN-γ has also been shown to upregulate CD40 on KC; triggering of CD40 by its natural T cell ligand gp39 induces ICAM-1 and Bcl-x$_L$ expression, as well as IL-8 secretion.[22] Thus, T cell/KC interaction via CD40/CD40L leads to the inhibition of KC apoptosis and the release of a cytokine which stimulates KC proliferation and induces neutrophil infiltration.

Activated KC also express BB-1 which, on binding to its ligand CD28, delivers a costimulatory signal required for optimal activation

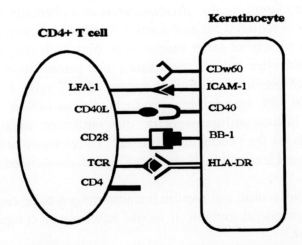

Fig. 8.3. Surface molecules mediating CD4⁺ T cell/KC interaction.

of T cells via the TCR/CD3 complex.[23] This would lead to more cytokine production by CD4$^+$ T cells which would further enhance upregulation of surface molecules on KC and therefore interaction between them.

CDw60 is also upregulated on lesional KC by the effects of cytokine released by T cells, in this case IL-13.[24] CDw60 acts as a costimulator for T cell activation, but the role of this molecule on psoriatic KC is unknown.

8.3.2 *Cytokines*

Various studies have shown that T cells from psoriatic skin lesions are capable of stimulating KC proliferation via the production of cytokines.[25,26] The predominant cytokine released by activated CD4$^+$ T cells, IFN-γ, is a potent inhibitor of KC proliferation when added alone. This apparent paradox can be explained by the decreased susceptibility of psoriatic KC to inhibition by IFN-γ,[27] and by the additional effects of other cytokines released by activated T cells such as IL-6 and IL-8.

Conversely, lesional but not normal epidermal cells release a mixture of cytokines, including IL-1β and IL-8, that potentiate T cell activation both via the TCR/CD3 complex and via other activating pathways (anti-CDw60).[28] In addition, KC produce cytokines such as IL-6, IL-8 and TGF-α which can have autocrine effects thus perpetuating the expansion of the psoriatic KC population.

8.4 Role of CD8$^+$ T Lymphocytes

Spontaneous resolution of guttate psoriatic lesions has been shown to coincide with the disappearance of activated CD4$^+$ T cells and epidermal recruitment and activation of CD8$^+$ T cells. In contrast, the epidermis of stable and long-lived CP lesions contain approximately equal numbers of activated CD4$^+$ and activated CD8$^+$ T cells. These findings suggest that at least two subpopulations of CD8$^+$ T cells may exist in psoriasis; one that switches off and a second that helps to maintain the psoriatic process, both of which could act via effects on CD4[+] T cell function. Indeed, two types of CD8[+] T cell with different cytokine patterns and functions, analogous to TH_1 and TH_2 cells, have recently been described.[29]

Suppression of antigen-activated CD4[+] T cells by CD8[+] T cells stimulated by SAg has been shown to result from their ability to induce CD4[+] T cell apoptosis via ligation of Fas.[30] Furthermore, although activated CD8[+] T cells expressed both Fas and FasL, they were themselves resistant to Fas-dependent apoptosis. It is conceivable that a similar mechanism may operate in spontaneously resolving guttate lesions whereby the activated CD4[+] T cells associated with initiation are deleted by activated CD8[+] T cells resulting in termination of the disease process.

In contrast, activated CD4[+] and activated CD8[+] T cells coexist in CP epidermis. Vβ analysis of epidermal CD8[+] T cells strongly suggests that the Vβ3[+] and Vβ13.1/3[+] T cell subsets recognise specific antigen presumably presented by MHC Class I-restricted APC, which could perhaps include KC. Furthermore, the same dominant T cell clones persisted over several months in individual patients implying an essential role for CD8[+] T cells in the psoriatic process. However, in contrast to CD4[+] T cells, CD8[+] T cells were unable to initiate the disease when injected into uninvolved psoriatic skin grafted onto SCID mice.[31] CP lesions may therefore be maintained by a subpopulation of CD8[+] T cells that require/send stimulatory signals from/to CD4[+] T cells.

The number of autoantigens recognised during an autoimmune response is not fixed. On the contrary, it expands both intra- and inter-molecularly over time, referred to as "epitope spreading". The response to these secondary determinants may involve antigen presentation by different MHC molecules than the response to the initial disease-inducing epitope. Thus, although initiation would be CD4[+] T cell mediated, expansion and perpetuation of the psoriatic process could involve both CD4[+] and CD8[+] T cells stimulated by secondary determinants presented by MHC Class II and Class I, respectively.

8.5 Site of Altered Gene Expression

Possible sites for the location of altered gene expression in psoriasis include the T lymphocyte, APC and KC, or a combination of these since this apppears to be a polygenic disease (see Chap. 1).

It is possible that CD4+ and/or CD8+ T cells specific for the putative autoantigen(s) in psoriasis also exist in normal individuals. However, the psoriatic autoimmune T cells may have a lower threshold of activation or produce a qualitatively and/or quantitatively different pattern of cytokines to that of their non-psoriatic counterparts.

A genetic alteration may influence APC processing and presentation in psoriasis so that streptococcal antigens are not eliminated. Thus, they accumulate in the skin where they stimulate T cells thus maintaining the psoriatic process (see above). Alternatively, there could be an altered binding affinity of psoriasis-related MHC molecules for streptococcal and/or autoantigen epitopes. The association of both MHC Class I and Class II alleles with psoriasis may be of relevance in this respect.

Perhaps the most likely site of altered gene expression in psoriasis is the KC. In contrast to normal KC, psoriatic KC have a decreased susceptibility to the inhibitory effects of IFN-γ, are stimulated by IFN-γ in cooperation with other growth factors produced by T cells, and conversely release a balance of cytokines that potentiate T cell activation. Furthermore, psoriatic KC appear to be resistant to apoptosis-inducing stimuli. One or all of these functional alterations could have a genetic basis.

8.6 Other Antigenic Triggers

Not all patients with psoriasis develop the acute, disseminated form of the disease or experience GAS-induced exacerbations of their skin lesions. Thus, evidently there must be other external triggers that induce or exacerbate psoriasis. This would not be incompatible with the proposed model since homology between human and foreign determinants is not confined to GAS, or even to bacteria.

Retroviruses have been implicated in psoriasis.[32] Furthermore, induction and/or worsening of psoriasis is striking in patients with AIDS. Mice transgenic for whole HIV proviral sequences develop scaling and epidermal hyperplasia similar to psoriasis,[33] hence suggesting that HIV could play a direct role in the pathogenesis. However, one or more of the various opportunistic infections associated with AIDS could also act as triggers.

It is possible that chronic plaques could be initiated by retroviruses and then maintained by autoreactive T cells recognising cross-reactive determinants in the skin. Alternatively, the ability of retroviruses to integrate permanently into the human genome, so called "endogenous retroviruses" may result in autoimmune disease via various mechanisms. Interestingly, a human endogenous retrovirus that encodes an MHC Class II-dependent SAg has been identified recently in patients with acute-onset type 1 diabetes.[34]

Recently human papillomavirus type 5 (HPV5), the virus associated with epidermodysplasia verruciformis, has been detected by a sensitive nested PCR technique in scrapings of lesional skin in approximately 90% of a large series of patients with psoriasis.[35] In contrast, no HPV5 DNA was detected in atopic dermatitis skin. Furthermore, HPV5-specific antibodies specific for the L1 capsid protein were found in approximately 25% of patients versus 2–5% of controls which included patients with atopic dermatitis, allograft recipients or patients with genital warts. These observations led Majewski et al.[36] to propose that HPV5 is the putative autoantigen recognised by oligoclonal epidermal CD8+ T cells in psoriatic lesions. However, since papillomavirus infection of KC is favoured by epidermal proliferation, it could be argued that infection is secondary to the hyperproliferative process in psoriasis and therefore represents a type of opportunistic infection.

Local skin infections with organisms such as *S.aureus* or *C.albicans* have been reported to exacerbate psoriasis. It has been postulated that this is mediated by the release of SAgs.[37] Furthermore, the presence of T cells reactive to *Pityrosporum* yeast in psoriatic scalp lesions suggests that organisms that form part of the normal skin flora may also act as triggers of the psoriatic process.[38]

The immunopathogenic pathway leading to the development of psoriasis remains to be fully elucidated. However, the model proposed here provides a basis for further studies which will enable the stimulating antigen(s) to be identified, and which will eventually determine whether psoriasis is an autoimmune disease or the result of a chronic streptococcal infection.

References

1. Baker B.S., Swain A.F., Fry L., Valdimarsson H. *Br.J.Dermatol.* **110** (1994), 555–564.
2. Valdimarsson H., Baker B.S., Jonsdottir I., Fry L. *Immunol.Today* **7** (1986), 256–259.
3. Lewis H. *et al. Br.J.Dermatol.* **129** (1993), 514–520.
4. Leung D.Y.M. *et al. J.Clin.Invest.* **96** (1995), 2106–2112.
5. Boehncke W.H. *Trends in Microbiol.* **485** (1996), 485–489.
6. Leung D.Y.M. *et al. J.Exp.Med.* **181** (1995), 747–753.
7. Menssen A. *et al. J.Immunol.* **155** (1995), 4078–4083.
8. Chang J.C.C. *et al. Proc.Natl.Acad.Sci. (USA)* **91** (1995), 9282–9286.
9. Chang J.C.C. *et al. Arch.Dermatol.* **133** (1997), 703–708.
10. Prinz J.C. *et al. Eur.J.Immunol.* **29** (1999), 3360–3368.
11. Steinle A., Reinhardt C., Jantzer P., Schendal D.J. *J.Exp.Med.* **181** (1995), 503–513.
12. Baker B.S. *et al. Br.J.Dermatol.* **128** (1993), 493–499.
13. Valdimarsson H. *et al. Immunol.Today* **145** (1995), 145–149.
14. Swerlick R.A., Cunningham M.W., Hall N.K. *J.Invest.Dermatol.* **87** (1986), 367–371.
15. McFadden J., Valdimarsson H., Fry L. *Br.J.Dermatol.* **125** (1991), 443–447.
16. Hunter I., Skerrow D. *Br.J.Dermatol.* **120** (1989), 363–370.
17. Sigmundsdottir H. *et al. Scand.J.Immunol.* **45** (1997), 688–697.
18. Gudmundsdottir A.S. *et al. Clin.Exp.Immunol.* **117** (1999), 580–586.
19. Pruksakorn S. *et al. Int.Immunol.* **6** (1994), 1235–1244.
20. Segal B.M., Klinman D.M., Shevach E.M. *J.Immunol.* **158** (1997), 5087–5090.

21. Yawalkar N. *et al. J.Invest.Dermatol.* **110** (1998), 665 (Abstract).
22. Goodman R.E. *et al. J.Immunol.* **152** (1994), 5189–5198.
23. Denfeld R.W. *et al. Eur.J.Immunol.* **26** (1996), 2329–2334.
24. Nickoloff B.J. *et al. J.Immunol.* **150** (1993), 2148–2159.
25. Skov L. *et al. Am.J.Pathol.* **150** (1997), 675–683.
26. Bata-Csorgo Z., Hammerberg C., Voorhees J.J., Cooper K.D. *J.Clin.Invest.* **95** (1995), 317–327.
27. Prinz J.C. *et al. Eur.J.Immunol.* **24** (1994), 593–598.
28. Baker B.S., Powles A.V., Valdimarsson H., Fry L. *Scand.J.Immunol.* **28** (1988), 735–740.
29. Chang E.Y. *et al. Arch.Dermatol.* **128** (1992), 1479–1485.
30. Mosmann T.R. and Sad S. *Immunol.Today* **17** (1996), 138–146.
31. Noble A., Pestano G.A., Cantor H. *J.Immunol.* **159** (1998), 559–565.
32. Nickoloff B.J. and Wrone-Smith T. *Am.J.Pathol.* **155** (1999), 145–158.
33. Iversen O.J., Nissen-Meyjer J., Dalen A.B. *Acta Pathol.Microbiol.Immunol. Scand.* **91** (1983), 413–417.
34. Leonard J.M. *et al. Science* **242** (1988), 1665–1670.
35. Conrad B. *et al. Cell* **90** (1997), 303–313.
36. Favre M. *et al. J.Invest.Dermatol.* **110** (1998), 311–317.
37. Majewski S., Favre M., Orth G., Jablonska S. *J.Invest.Dermatol.* **111** (1998), 541–542.
38. Leung D.Y.M., Walsh P., Storno R., Norris D.A. *J.Invest.Dermatol.* **100** (1993), 225–228.
39. Baker B.S. *et al. Br.J.Dermatol.* **136** (1997), 319–325.

Index